T0258470

CRAVING EARTH

Craving Earth

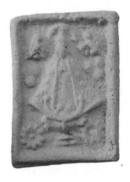

Understanding Pica

The Urge to Eat Clay, Starch, Ice, and Chalk

Sera L. Young

COLUMBIA UNIVERSITY PRESS　NEW YORK

Columbia University Press
Publishers Since 1893
New York   Chichester, West Sussex
Copyright © 2011 Sera L. Young
All rights reserved
Library of Congress Cataloging-in-Publication Data
Young, Sera L.
Craving earth : understanding pica : the urge to eat clay, starch,
ice, and chalk / Sera L. Young.
p. ; cm.
Includes bibliographical references and index.
ISBN 978-0-231-14608-1 (cloth : alk. paper) —
ISBN 978-0-231-51789-8
(ebook)
1. Pica (Pathology)   I. Title.
[DNLM: 1. Pica—ethnology   2. Pica—history.
3. Food Habits—psychology. WM 175]
GN408.Y68 2011
613.2—dc22
2010031789

Columbia University Press books are printed on permanent and durable
acid-free paper.
This book is printed on paper with recycled content.
Printed in the United States of America
c 10 9 8 7 6 5 4 3 2 1
References to Internet Web sites (URLs) were accurate at the time of writing.
Neither the author nor Columbia University Press is responsible for URLs that may
have expired or changed since the manuscript was prepared.

The image that appears on the title page and at each chapter heading is a
bendito, a sacred clay tablet imprinted with an image of the Virgin Mary.
Catholics and others have ascribed healing, fertility, and protective
powers to the ingestion of such tablets. This tablet was kindly provided
by Professor Louis Grivetti.

For Stella, the first young Lucks

Contents

List of Illustrations

Preface

"EVERY DAY, twice a day, I take a chunk of earth from this wall and, well, I eat it."

Had I understood Mama Sharifa* correctly?

We were sitting on a woven palm mat, in the only shade in her sun-baked yard, on a tiny Zanzibari island called Pemba. There were three of us: Mama Sharifa, Biubwa (my research assistant), and me. Our backs were against the dirt wall of her outdoor kitchen, our legs stretched out in front of us, discussing the things she eats during pregnancy.

With raised eyebrows, I looked to Biubwa to confirm that I had indeed understood her Swahili. Biubwa nodded. "Yes, she is saying she eats earth."

"But why?" I asked.

Mama Sharifa bent at the waist as much as her pregnant belly would allow to idly slap at a fly on her ankle. Then she looked away from us. "I just eat it, that's all." Her pink and orange *kanga*, a light cotton cloth frequently worn as a head covering, shifted over her shoulder and obscured her face, and I feared she would say no more on the matter.

But after a long pause, her arm reached out from under her kanga. She turned toward us, plucked a chunk of earth from the highest part of the

---

*Throughout the book, names have been changed to preserve anonymity.

wall she could reach, and displayed it in her open palm. I looked from the chunk of earth in her hand to her face and then back to her hand.

I smiled at her and repeated my question. "But why, Mama?"

She was giggling by then, out of what I've come to recognize as a combination of embarrassment and sheer inability to answer this question. She brushed at some dust on her long skirt, then stared off into the distance again. And then she locked eyes with me.

"I don't know. I really don't know. I just do it."

She offered the earth to me, and I took it. First I smelled it. Then I touched it to the tip of my tongue. Then I nibbled into it. It tasted bland, like old air. But after I swallowed, my tongue felt different, dried out, as from the astringency of tea that has been brewed for too long. A few grains of sand remained in my mouth long after we had moved on to other topics.

But for the rest of that research period on Pemba, and for the many that have since followed, I learned as much about earth-eating as I could. I asked pregnant women about their motivations. I quizzed fellow passengers on buses. I asked the old men drinking Arabic coffee at dusk. I probed nurses in the antenatal clinics. What other non-food items did people crave? Did all pregnant women have these cravings? Was it only pregnant women? Did anyone know why they did it? Where did the idea to eat these things come from? Is it some sort of religious phenomenon? Which earth is the stuff for eating? However, my pestering raised more questions than it answered.

During another interview that summer, the responsibility for understanding pica was unexpectedly shifted to me. I asked Mama Khadija, the second wife of a traditional healer, if she knew why people eat earth.

Uhh, no, I don't know.
Do you have any *ideas* about why some people sometimes eat it?
No.
Are you sure?
Yes!
Not even one idea?

This time, she didn't reply but just looked at me, smiling slightly, shaking her head as one does with an incorrigible child. I sheepishly apologized for asking so many questions. But she then said something that changed the trajectory of my academic pursuits. She pointed at my clipboard and recorder and said, "Since you're the researcher, why don't *you* find out and tell us?"

And with that, dear reader, our adventures with pica begin.

CRAVING EARTH

PART ONE

All About Pica

CHAPTER ONE

What on Earth?

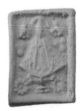**MAMA SHARIFA** eats chunks from the earthen wall of her outdoor kitchen in Zanzibar, while in Washington, D.C., Pat crunches through a ten-pound bag of ice from 7-Eleven every day. In New Delhi, Simran starts her morning with a handful of uncooked rice, and in Mississippi, Tanya eats Argo cornstarch, but only after her husband has gone to work. In Guatemala, Carlita nibbles little blocks of clay with a Virgin Mary pressed into them, while in California, D'angela buys ten boxes of chalkboard chalk for snacking whenever she can get to a Walmart. What is the common denominator? These are all instances of **pica** (see Glossary).

Pica is the scientific term for the craving and subsequent consumption of non-food items.[1] It's not an acronym, or an abbreviation, or a famous physician's last name. *Pica pica* is the genus and species of the common magpie (fig. 1.1). Magpies are frequently seen with all sorts of items in their beaks, from chewing gum wrappers to wire hangers. Because of their attraction to sparkly objects, they were thought to be birds with an indiscriminate appetite. (As it turns out, they don't swallow these items; they build their nests with them.) By analogy, the human condition of desiring non-food items was given the name "pica" in the sixth century (Aetius of Amida/Ricci 1542 [1950]:20). I use the term *pica* to mean the craving and

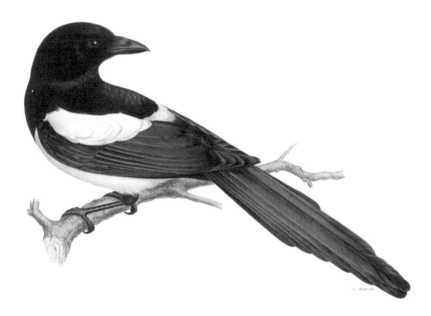

FIGURE 1.1

The magpie, *Pica pica*. Drawing by Wilhelm von Wright (1810–1887), from *Svenska fåglar, efter naturen och på sten ridade* (*see* http://commons.wikipedia.org/wiki/File:Pica_pica).

purposive consumption of items that the consumer does not consider to be food for more than a month (Young 2010).

Pica is not the only name for this behavior, however. Eating non-food items has been referred to in many ways in the two thousand years that people have been writing about it. Some terms are very arcane. *Citta*, for example, is a term that Galen used for pica; it is Greek for ivy, but may be a misspelling of *kitta*, which is Greek for magpie or jay (Weiss-Amer 1993). Other general terms that have been used as synonyms for pica include cachexia (Liebault 1598), cachexia Africana (Chisholm 1799), chthonophagia (Dors [Dons] 1838), hapsicoria (Motherby 1785), mal d'estomac (Thibault de Chanvalon 1761), malacia (Liebault 1598), and paroroexia (Ruddock 1924).

Pica is a general term, and in modern medical literature eating non-food items is frequently referred to in more specific ways. Names for specific types of pica generally have Greek origins. They combine the names of specific substances, e.g., "geo" (earth), "amylon" (starch), and "pagos" (ice), with "phagein" (to eat), thus yielding **geophagy**,[2] **amylophagy**, and **pagophagy** (Coltman 1969).[3]

4

The Pica Substances

Earth is the most commonly craved substance, but it is far from the only one. In fact, the list of pica substances is very long. In roughly descending order of frequency, it also includes cornstarch, ice (if consumed in large quantities), chalk, charcoal, ash, flour, newspaper, toilet paper, used coffee grounds, baby powder, and paint chips. While this list may seem highly heterogeneous, there is one commonality. With the exception of ice, all of these substances are dry, powdery, and adsorptive (see **adsorption**), and most of them are rather crunchy.

Just as we now know that the magpie's appetite is not indiscriminant—those non-food items in their beaks are housing materials, not lunch—pica cravings are not indiscriminant, either. People regularly go out of their way to obtain items that have the precise odor, texture, and taste they desire, as you'll see in the following descriptions of the three most frequently craved pica substances.

Earth (geophagy)

Humans have been consuming earth for a very long time. There is good evidence to suggest that we were even eating it two million years ago, when we *Homo sapiens* were still *Homo habilis* (Clark 2001:659–62; see also Appendix A, this volume).[4] Earth is consumed in many forms and comes from many sources including mud from a riverbed, broken bits of pottery, earth clods found among dry pinto beans. The amount consumed daily varies, but quantities of 20–40 g are typically reported (Geissler et al. 1997; Luoba et al. 2005; Saathoff et al. 2002; Young et al. 2010b), Most of the earth consumed is rich in clay (Young 2010); although clays may seem unremarkable, they have amazing properties that are discussed at length in chapter 3.

But not just any earth will do. People go to extreme lengths to obtain the earth of their heart's desire. They may be secretive about the whereabouts of their clay pit (Silverman and Perkens 1966), walk many miles to the site with "good dirt" (Dickens and Ford 1942), tussle with the cattle who are also eating "their" clay (Hunter 1993), and implore relatives to mail boxes of clay when they move to a place with unappetizing soil (1967; Dickens and Ford 1942; Frate 1984). The smoothest soils (i.e., those high in clay content) are the most sought after, from the Arctic (Richardson 1851:191) to the Amazon (von Humboldt et al. 1821, pt. 2, pp. 639–64), and everywhere in between. Sandy soils and soils high in dark organic material, called **humus**, are typically avoided.

The smell of earth is an important criterion for soil selection the world over over (e.g., Forsyth and Benoit 1989; Hooper and Mann 1906; McIntyre 2000). The earth's scent after rain, called *petrichor* (Bear and Thomas 1964), is a particularly important indicator of its suitability.[5] During ethnographic interviews, women's mouths would literally water as they described to me the appealing smell of freshly moistened earth.

Another criterion for geophagists is that their dirt be "clean." Most earth for consumption is collected from places where animals do not tread (and therefore cannot defecate), such as from areas high up on a wall or the interior of a well; others insure the hygiene of their earth by drying and/or heating it, either in the sun or over open flame (Young et al. 2007).

One of the stories that best illustrates the acuity of geophagists' selectivity involves a geophagic wife, a devoted husband anxious to avoid trouble, and police surveillance in Memphis, Tennessee (Finger 1993). The wife sent her husband to get her some clay from her favorite riverbank. She did not want to go because police had been staking out the site, suspicious of the many small holes dug into the bank. But she just *had* to have some. He dutifully left the house and returned with a bag of earth for her. When she opened it, she knew immediately that it was not from her favorite riverbank spot. She sent him right back out for earth from the stakeout riverbank.

Earth-eating is far more common than just a few cases here and there. Estimates range from <0.01% among pregnant Danish women (Mikkelsen et al. 2006), to 5.2% among pregnant Pembans, to 56% among pregnant women in coastal Kenya (Geissler et al. 1998b); Appendices B and C summarize studies of the prevalence of different types of pica among representative samples of pregnant women and children, respectively.

Commoditization is a great indicator of demand, and yes, geophagic earth is now for sale. In fact, there is enough demand across the United States that Sam's General Store, a shop in White Plains, Georgia, that sells geophagic earth, has established an online presence (http://whitedirt .samsbiz.com/). They sell earth in two-pound increments, marked as "a novelty item" (probably to avoid any lawsuits). And just in case you are worried about what the postman may think, their deliveries arrive discretely in unmarked cardboard boxes.

Sam's General Store sells **kaolin**, which many geophagists consider to be the most desirable type of clay. However, there are many types of earth eaten, and almost as many names for it. For example, on Pemba Island, where I first learned about geophagy, people eat four types of earth. Their

6

Swahili names are *udongo, ufue, vitango pepeta* (also known as *vitango mlima*) and *mchanga*. In other places, the variety of geophagic soils is even greater (e.g., Vermeer 1971).

And where does geophagy happen? We know for sure that it occurs on all six inhabited continents (Hooper and Mann 1906). Our best information about the worldwide distribution of geophagy comes from ethnographic literature, i.e., reports from anthropologists, missionaries, and explorers. I have assimilated data from 367 such reports of geophagy, and it is clearly ubiquitous (fig. 1.2). The methods for this analysis are described in chapter 2. The worldwide distribution of pica is discussed in greater detail in chapter 9.

Raw Starch (amylophagy)

These days, it's easy to think of starches as a food group to avoid, thanks to the demonization of carbohydrates by the infamous Atkins diet. But take a look at any USDA food pyramid and you'll see that starches—rice, pasta, breads, and tortillas—ought to provide the bulk of our calories. Uncooked starches, too, have a place in our daily lives, although they have little to offer us calorically.[6] Even so, they play a role in our cuisine. They thicken Thanksgiving gravies, give lightness to Christmas shortbread, and prevent powdered sugar from caking.

Raw starches have another function, one that is germane to pica: they sate extraordinarily strong cravings. Until a few decades ago, raw starch was available in most grocery stores in two different products, both of which were attractive to amylophagists. There was cornstarch, mostly used for thickening foods, and there was laundry starch. In the 1960s, before the convenience of spray starch and the magic of wrinkle-free fabrics, if you wanted unwrinkled shirts you needed laundry starch. Back then, laundry starch, which can be made from corn, wheat, or rice starches, was sold in big chunks. When it came time to do the starching, these chunks would be dissolved in warm water, laundered clothes would be dipped into the solution and, once dry, they would be ironed. Besides nicely crisping your collars, it was handy for preventing stains: daily grime would bind to the starch rather than to the fibers of the cloth, making it easy to rinse out.

Many women seeking substitutes for earth that is no longer available have turned to starch as a replacement (e.g., Associated Press 1988; Hertz 1947; McIntyre 2000; Vermeer and Frate 1975). This was particularly common in the mid-1900s among black women who moved from the southern

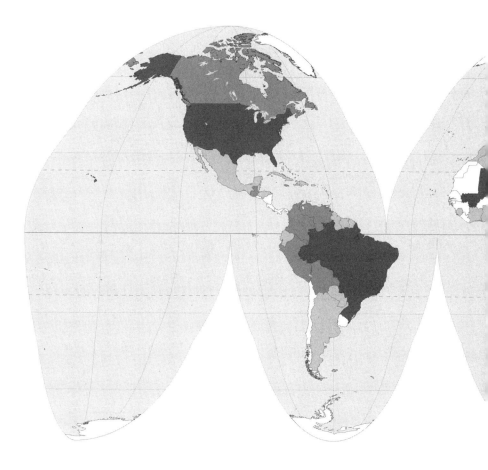

FIGURE 1.2
Distribution of 367 ethnographic reports of geophagy, by country (based on the Pica Literature Database). Map created by Geographical Techniques (www.geotechmap.com).

United States to industrial areas like Chicago and Detroit, where the earth they desired was not available. A photograph of a Washington, D.C., resident, in which she and her giggling young son pop chunks of starch in their mouths, appeared in a 1967 *Time* magazine with the caption: "As good as clay any day."[7] (Even Argo's cornstarch packaging suggests how its starch may be substituted for clay, albeit not for human consumption. On the outside of some Argo starch packages, there is a recipe for "Play Clay" in which Argo is the main ingredient.)

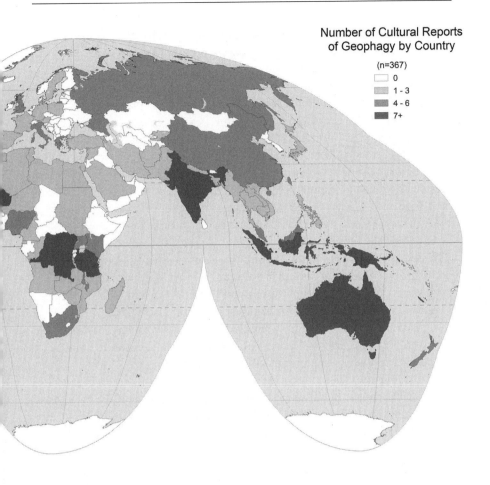

Number of Cultural Reports
of Geophagy by Country

(n=367)
☐ 0
▨ 1 - 3
▨ 4 - 6
■ 7+

For many women, though, starch is not a mere substitute; it is *the* most desirable substance. An enormous variety of raw starches are craved and consumed around the world, including uncooked rice (Giudicelli and Combes 1992; Kettaneh et al. 2005; Posner et al. 1957; Roselle 1970; Young et al. 2010a), wheat, cassava, and rice flours (Kraemer 2002; Levacher 1840; Ward and Kutner 1999), and raw starchy vegetables (tubers) including potatoes and cassava (Johnson and Stephens 1982; Libnoch 1984). However, at least in the United States, cornstarch once reigned over them all.

That reign has been curtailed, due in large part to the untiring efforts of Dr. Gerald Deas. Dr. Deas is an animated, hands-on physician who still makes house calls and cares seriously about public health: think Cliff Huxtible meets Florence Nightingale. In the 1960s, when he was interning in a Brooklyn obstetrics clinic, he noticed that a lot of black women, "maybe 99 percent," were eating starch (Cleaton 1983; Day 2000). Dr. Deas explained to me that "in those days, starch was typically stocked in the snack aisle of the grocery store, along with cookies and candy." He, like many, believed that eating starch caused iron deficiency, and so felt compelled to reduce its prevalence. He was also concerned about the weight gain associated with eating large quantities of starch: one box of cornstarch contains 1,680 Calories, and some women eat as many as three boxes in a day.[8]

So, Dr. Deas became a one-man campaign to educate women about the dangers of starch-eating. He helped to produce pamphlets with catchy, community-friendly slogans that were distributed by the National Urban League: "If you eat laundry starch, you'll become a stiff"; "Eating laundry starch from a box is as nutritious as eating rocks"; and "The main thing is what is that package of starch doing to your package [fetus]?" He wrote columns in local newspapers and appeared on radio shows and news broadcasts to discuss the dangers of starch-eating.

His public-awareness campaign efforts paid off tangibly in the reform of the packaging and marketing of starch (fig. 1.3). In 1977 the director of public relations at Best Foods (which produces Argo starch) sent him a letter stating that "the next order of their packaging material will have 'Not recommended for food use' prominently displayed on the front panel." Several years later, Best Foods made a second modification to Argo starch, one that morphed it into the product found on grocery store shelves today: they began to sell Argo starch in a powderized form. This was a significant blow to pica enthusiasts.[9] The hard chunks of starch were extremely appealing both because of their crunchy texture and the handiness of stowing them in a purse or innocent-looking paper bag (Edwards et al. 1959; Richardson 2002).

Although Dr. Deas has done much to halt **amylophagy** in the United States, there is evidence that it continues today. Currently on YouTube there is a fascinating video of Suerenity, a very pretty and very pregnant woman, eating cornstarch straight from the box. And if you join the Cornstarch Discussion Group on Yahoo! Groups, you will see it is filled with women "freaking out" over their "addiction to this starch." Here's a typical response to a new member who introduced herself by explaining she had been addicted to cornstarch and baby powder for the last fifteen years.

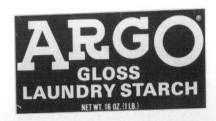

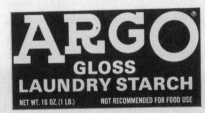

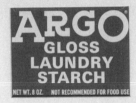

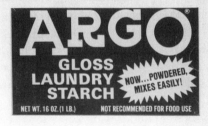

FIGURE 1.3
The evolution of the Argo starch label (Cleaton 1983). The top image is the original label on Argo laundry starch. The middle label features a warning in the lower right-hand corner, added in 1977. The third image reflects further modification: Best Foods' decision to sell their starch in powdered form, rather than as chunks. Images graciously provided by Dr. Gerald Deas.

"Honey we all eat starch, or baby powder, or baking soda . . . some kind of something strange in this group lol. You be reading a lot of stories about those things. I personally love starch and have been eating it for 10 yrs now. . . . . WELCOME HOME LOL!!!!"

A number of population-level studies of amylophagy from the last few decades corroborate these anecdotes (cf. Appendix B). In a study among 361 rural Mississippian women, 39% had eaten laundry starch (Ferguson and Keaton 1950). In East Texas, one-third of the 150 women interviewed had eaten starch or clay during at least one pregnancy (Taylor 1979), and of nearly 1,000 randomly selected pregnant women in Chicago, 35% had eaten starch (Keith et al. 1968). In our own study of 2,368 pregnant Pembans done in 2004, 36% had eaten uncooked rice in their current pregnancy (Young et al. 2010a).

The amount of starch typically eaten has not been well measured. There are reports of women eating several boxes of cornstarch a day (1967; Allan and Woodruff 1963; Roselle 1970; Warshauer 1966), but on Pemba, for example, the mean amount of raw rice consumed daily was only 26 grams, less than a palmful (Young et al. 2010a).

Ice (pagophagy)

Ice is another common pica substance. Now, don't think that you practice pica because you crunch the ice in your glass of Coke; a few cubes here and there is not pica. Pagophagists are people who *love* ice, *crave* ice, and *need* ice, and consequently, eat a whole lot of it. How much is a lot? The amount of ice they consume per day ranges from several glasses (Reynolds et al. 1968), to several ice cube trays (Brown and Dyment 1972; Moss et al. 1974; Osman et al. 2005), to several bowls (Sontag et al. 2001; Speirs and Jacobson 1976), to several pounds (Coltman 1969; Cooksey 1995; Haanen and Tan-tjiong 1982).

While the written evidence of **pagophagy** indicates it is younger than geophagy, it too is centuries old. The oldest written description was authored by a French Royal physician in the seventeenth century (Riverius et al. 1663). In his concisely named oeuvre "The practice of physick wherein is plainly set forth the nature, cause, differences, and several sorts of signs: Together with the cure of all diseases in the body of man. With many additions in several places never printed before," Riverius described the *desiderata* of those with pica:

Some require sowr things, sharp, bitter, and very cold, so that they are delighted with the continual use of unripe Fruits, Vinegar, Snow, Juyce of Lemmons, Pomegranates, and Oranges, cold Water, Snow, Ice and the like. Others desire Earthy, Dry, and burnt things, as Cloves, Cinnamon, Nutmegs, and other Spices, Salt-Ashes, Chalk, and the like. (Bk. 9, ch. 3)

Pagophagists are as picky about their ice as geophagists are about their earth. Once a person finds exactly the ice they like, they are hooked, returning to the restaurant or party store or laboratory icemaker again and again, sometimes multiple times per day. On icechewing.com, a Web site dedicated to the joys and difficulties of chewing lots of ice, the general consensus is that the ice at Sonic fast-food drive-ins is superior:

Hi I am visiting this site for the first time as I sit here at work doing what I am notorious for . . . chewing ice. This is the first post I saw and I am cracking up! Sonic has the best ice on earth aside from what I call rabbit turd ice. I know that sounds gross but I am guessing if you love to chew ice like I do you know what I mean . . . you know that ice that is soft and almost cylindrical in shape. Well anyhoo glad I found this site. Hopeful knowing there are others out there like myself I won't feel so strange about it. :lol:

OHHHHH, dat Sonic Ice goes so hard!!! I love Sonic Ice, LOL, I thought I was the only one but I buy it by the bags not cups!!! It costs $2.12.

In fact, there are so many fans of Sonic Ice that it even has its own Facebook page, with 208,554 fans. One quote on Sonic Ice's wall: "I NEVER join these things but I really DO love Sonic Ice!!"

The lengths people go to, especially pregnant women, to obtain the ice they crave can be astounding. They drive for hours or sleep very little so that they can crunch their ice away from the prying eyes of their family. One woman even bought the machine they use at Sonic (a Scotsman MDT2C12 Touchfree Air Cooled Cubelet Ice Maker/Dispenser) to have in her home: "Found on e-bay, paid $2250 for the thing." Short of purchasing an industrial icemaker, there are other tactics to ensure a steady ice or frost supply: frequently borrowing trays of ice cubes from many neighbors; leaving the door of a deep freezer open a crack so that frost continuously forms; and sending boyfriends and husbands out for ice, even in snowstorms (Cooksey 1995).

"A devouring passion"

You may have noticed that one common feature among these picas is strong cravings. To say that geophagists "eat earth" does not convey the frequently imperative nature of their drive. In fact, the desire for pica substances is so strong that those who have not experienced pica have long equated the strength of these cravings with those for tobacco, alcohol, and drugs.

In Jamaica in 1788: "Their attachment [to earth] is greater than even that of dram drinkers to their pernicious liquor" (Hunter 1788:310).

In Georgia in 1840: "From the oldest to little children, [they] are as much addicted to the eating of clay as some communities are to the use of tobacco and snuff" (Burke 1978 [1871]:79).

In England in 1842: "Powerfully do the morbid appetites enslave a large portion of mankind—from the opium of China to the tobacco of Virginia, and from the beer of England and the whisky of Ireland to the clay of Carolina" (Buckingham 1842:551).

In India in 1906: "The uncontrollable craving for this [earth] is like the opium or alcohol habit, and the ravenous symptoms and anxiety in the faces and actions of the eaters are similar to those found in the devotees of one or other of these vices" (Hooper and Mann 1906:264).

Those who actually engage in pica use similarly strong terms to characterize their cravings; sometimes the language used to discuss pica is exactly that used to describe illicit drug use. For example, one of the Swahili terms used in Pemba to discuss pica is *vileo*, which is the same word used to describe addiction to cigarettes, alcohol, or hard drugs. A Washington, D.C., woman told a reporter for *Time* magazine that, "When I'm pregnant, it's just like taking dope" (1967). And such language is echoed in the Yahoo! Cornstarch Discussion Group:

I had been 2 days clean and went over to a friends house. I had told this friend that I did cornstarch and was getting off it. They wanted me to finish this box, it only had a little in it, just to see how I do this. [. . .] I finished off the starch (it wasn't much) and have been craving that taste ever since!!!! I even drove miles out of my way to go to this store they were talking about. It wasn't there. MAN I WANT THAT TASTE AGAIN!!!!

Given this strong desire, it should be no surprise that people have a very hard time ceasing their pica behavior. Pica literature is peppered with phrases like "nothing is sufficient to prevent them from indulging their morbid cravings" (Imray 1843). Descriptions of the punishment meted out to slaves who engaged in pica make it clear that even terrible physical punishment, including whippings and iron masks, was no deterrent (cf. chapter 6).

Difficulties with stopping are also a feature of 21st-century pica behavior. In Laos, threats of arrest did not cause the cessation of geophagy (Rowles-Sewing 1981). Women in the Yahoo! Cornstarch Discussion Group spend a lot of time sharing advice on techniques for curbing behavior; promises to God, extraordinary weight gain, and threats of divorce are insufficient to dissuade them. Pica today remains the "devouring passion" it was described as a century ago (Galt 1872). For this reason, the phrase "craving and purposive consumption" is an important part of the definition of pica.

Who Does Pica?

We know that people around the world engage in pica; at this very moment there are hundreds of thousands of people experiencing cravings to eat all kinds of non-food items. But there are some segments of the population more likely to engage in pica than others. Pregnant women easily comprise the largest proportion of consumers, while children form the second largest group. (Detailed discussions of populations more likely to engage in pica are found in chapters 6, 8, and 9.)

Pregnant Women

Pica is so overwhelmingly associated with pregnancy that in some places it is synonymous with pregnancy. For example, when a senior government physician in Malawi was asked if village women ate clay in pregnancy, she smiled: "It would be very surprising if pregnant women in Malawi did not eat clay. That's how you know when you are pregnant!" (Hunter 1993:75). In Nigeria, "the association of this custom with pregnancy reaches the point that women note axiomatically that if a woman is observed to eat clay, she must be pregnant" (Vermeer 1966:200).

This association with pregnancy is both ubiquitous and very old. Hippocrates (460–377 B.C.E.) is responsible for the first written record of geophagy, and in it he specifically identifies pregnant women. "If a pregnant woman would like to eat earth or charcoal, and then eats it, the child that enters this world will be marked on its head from these substances" (Hippocrates 1853:487).

One of the most luscious passages about pica during pregnancy is found in the *Raghuvamsha*, a thirteenth-century epic Indian poem that traces the genealogy of dynasty of warrior kings (Kale 1997; see also Appendix D for more pica references in literature). Queen Sudakshina became a geophagist during her pregnancy; she had "set her heart upon clay in preference to all other objects of taste" (Canto III, nos. 3 & 4). Although the king didn't like the smell of "her mouth, fragrant with clay," his aversion to her earthy breath was overshadowed by her alluring pregnant body. "As days rolled on, her two breasts, growing exceedingly plump, and with nipples black all round, far surpassed the loveliness of a couple of well-formed lotus buds with black bees perched upon them" (Canto III, no. 8).

There is also plenty of scientific evidence that pica is associated with pregnancy. Biomedical studies of the prevalence of pica in dozens of antenatal populations in North America, South America, Africa, and Europe have shown again and again that pregnant women regularly engage in pica (cf. Appendix B).

Children

Young children are the second most likely to purposively consume non-food substances, although there are far fewer anecdotal reports of their pica behavior than for pregnant women (Young 2010). Please note, pica among children does *not* include exploratory mouthing behaviors. To be considered pica, children must actively seek out clay, paper, chalk, dirt, termite hills, etc. For this reason, pica cannot possibly occur until after children are over two years of age. There are also far fewer clinic-based studies of the prevalence of pica among schoolchildren, but the few that have been conducted suggest ranges from 1.7% (among children in upstate New York) (Marchi and Cohen 1990) to 74.4% (among Zambian schoolchildren) (Nchito et al. 2004). All epidemiologic studies on the prevalence of pica in children are presented in Appendix C.

Animals

Although this book is about human behavior, geophagy in the animal kingdom is widespread enough to merit mention. It is important to know that non-food consumption is not only a human activity because it suggests that there is some benefit to the phenomenon among us human animals: wild animals almost always behave in ways that are likely to promote their survival.

The below-referenced instances of geophagy among animals do *not* include visits to salt deposits or the practice of licking the earth in areas with high salt concentrations. In such instances, the motive is clear: the animal is seeking sodium. By geophagy, I am referring to animals who actively seek out the earth itself, in the absence of sodium. And many, many species do this.

There are some wonderful review articles about geophagy in nonhuman primates (Krishnamani and Mahaney 2000), terrestrial mammals (Hui 2004; Klaus and Schmid 1998), herbivores (Kreulen 1985), and birds (Diamond et al. 1999). And there are an even greater number of scientific articles detailing observations among individual species. For example, along the border between Kenya and Uganda, elephants have excavated deep caves in their quest for earth (Houston et al. 2001; Lundberg et al. 2006). In Yellowstone, grizzly bears consume soil in early spring and late summer (Mattson et al. 1999). Smaller mammals do, too, including hindgut herbivores like rhinoceros, zebra, and horse; ruminants like giraffe, kudu, eland, antelope, water buffalo, and duiker; and small herbivores like tapir, grouse, rabbit, squirrel, koala, and tortoise (Barlow 2000).

But Why?

By now, you must be wondering why all these human and nonhuman animals are eating earth and starch and ice, given the hassle, the cost, and the pleas not to. That is the exact question I propose to answer in this book. It's a tough one; after all, scientists continue to debate its function, if any, after two thousand years of study. But given how widespread the practice is, especially among some of the most vulnerable segments of our society (pregnant women and children), it's one worth answering.

In the pursuit of an answer, we will scoot through the history of medicine, touch on some of the world's greatest literature, and enter the guts and minds of pregnant women, encountering armchair anthropologists,

Nobel laureates, and tortured slaves along the way. We will unravel royal intrigues, become acquainted with several pantheons, and test a number of scientific hypotheses using a range of data, from randomized clinical trials to mineralogical analyses. But best of all, through the concurrent study of culture and biology, we will make scientific progress by making sense of some very chaotic data.

To begin, I will outline the biocultural framework, the perspective I have used to study pica (chapter 2). You may want to skim it if you are reading only for content about pica, but it does introduce some useful concepts that are peppered throughout the rest of the book. The rest of part I (chapters 3–5) further contextualizes pica by dealing broadly with humans' use of non-food substances. In chapter 3 ("Medicine You Can Walk On: The Amazing Properties of Clays"), I describe the many ways that pica substances have been used both internally and topically to heal a range of ailments from the "bitings of venemous poison-outcasting beasts" to explosive diarrhea. Chapter 4 ("Religious Geophagy: Sacredness You Can Swallow") details the uses of earth in religion: Christianity, Islam, Hinduism, and hoodoo folk magic. Both chapters 3 and 4 deal with geophagy that is not pica; these are not instances of craving earth, but provide an important context for the practices of pica. Chapter 5 ("Poisons and Pathogens") presents the darker side of pica and describes the harm that pica substances have been associated with. With this background, you will have the knowledge necessary for the second part of the book, which evaluates the many explanations of pica.

Part II deals uniquely with the etiology, or causes, of pica and opens with chapter 6 ("Dismissal and Damnation"), about the historical perspectives on the causes of pica among six groups who have most frequently been documented as engaging in pica. For each group, I suggest why such conclusions can be rejected.

Chapters 7, 8, and 9 are the most data-rich, scientific chapters of the book. They describe and evaluate the three most plausible hypotheses about the physiological functions of pica: that it is a response to hunger; that it is a response to a **micronutrient** deficiency such as iron or calcium; and that it occurs to protect against harm from toxins and pathogens. By chapter 10 ("Putting the Pica Pieces Together"), you'll be very knowledgeable about pica.

As you read, you may want to refer to the glossary and appendices at the end of the book. Four of the appendices summarize different types of biomedical studies on pica. Additionally, there are two more that attempt to organize different types of information on pica: a timeline of notable moments in the history of pica and instances of pica in literature.

One proviso: this is not an arcane volume that requires intimate knowledge of nutritional, soil, or biomedical sciences. After several years of studying pica, I find it too fascinating a topic to address only in academic journals. Thus, I have sought to write a book that is both accessible and pleasurable for people with a variety of backgrounds. In fact, you don't even need to have heard of pica to enjoy this book. I've worked hard to distill and translate the jargon from thousands of sources so that the only prerequisite to reading this book is a healthy dose of curiosity. Of course, if you would like greater scientific detail than I provide here, I would encourage you to track down some of the hundreds of references with which this book is laced. Finally, if you have specific questions about pica or want to share your own personal experiences with it, feel free to contact me at sera@younglucks.com or www.serayoung.org.

CHAPTER TWO

A Biocultural Approach

A Holistic Way to Study Pica

Among all the curious perversions of taste existing in various
parts of the world, there are few so peculiar or so apparently
unaccountable as that of eating earth. Were the habit not very
widely extended over the word, it would perhaps hardly be worth
any extended investigations but it is found among the peoples of
every continent, and apparently of almost every race.

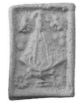 SO BEGINS the 1906 ethnography "Earth-Eating and the
Earth-Eating Habit in India" (Hooper and Mann 1906:250).
It is a fitting quote to open this chapter because it highlights
why geophagy (and pica in general) merits "extended investigations" or the careful thought process that is outlined in this
chapter. If pica were some seldom seen anomaly, like a puppy
with five legs or octuplets, we could afford to expend less brainpower on it.
But because it is found "among the peoples of every continent," especially
among the most vulnerable segments, and is associated with both positive
and negative health outcomes, we cannot afford to marvel and move on.

Pica, however, is hard to study; to this day, scientists continue to wrestle
with its causes and consequences. Actually, it's even hard to spell: the word
geophagy cost 12-year-old Katie Kuba the national spelling bee champion-
ship in 1995 (Associated Press 1995). The purpose of this chapter is to
make the examination of pica slightly easier by presenting a framework for
its study.

I have used a biocultural approach to respond to Mama Khadija's re-
quest to tell her what causes pica (cf. preface). In this chapter, I first define
what the biocultural approach is and then outline its five general principles.
The second part discusses the methods my collaborators and I have used
for gathering biocultural data on pica.

The Biocultural Perspective

Clearly, it's necessary to look at biology as well as culture when we study pica; pica could be attributed to biological needs, cultural beliefs, or both. But what, specifically, are "biology" and "culture"? You could line a library with books dedicated to defining them. Combine the two words together, and the possible definitions increase many-fold (Roth 2004). The number of definitions increases yet again as more disciplines are canvassed. If you could corral a dozen anthropologists, psychologists, demographers, and biologists into a room and ask them to emerge with a definition of biocultural, you are likely to be offered thirteen definitions instead. In short, no one can quite agree what **biocultural** means, and there are both biological anthropologists and cultural anthropologists who strongly dislike this term. For this reason, any definition I propose puts me in dangerous territory. Still, it's worth mapping the components of one definition of biocultural to see how regard for both biology and culture can shape our understanding of pica.

My description of "biocultural" draws heavily on the ecological model that nutritional anthropologists Drs. Norge Jerome, Randy Kandel, and Gretel Pelto penned in 1980 (Jerome et al. 1980), with only a few modifications (Young 2002; Young and Pelto 2006). Figure 2.1 is a graphical representation of how we can think about humans interacting with cultural and biological domains through their linkage with diet. The various domains are indicated by boxes, while arrows indicate interaction between domains. Although aspects of society are not as easily compartmentalized as the figure implies, it is a heuristic tool that is useful for drawing attention to and organizing the complexities of the context of human behavior.

This framework spans both biology and culture. It encompasses the physical environment in which we have matured as individuals and evolved as a species (upper right), and the biological functioning of our bodies (center). It includes cultural institutions at the macro-level of society (e.g., history, economic opportunities, and power relations: upper left), as well as at the micro-level (i.e., household and family dynamics: lower left). Ideational beliefs (center bottom) and technological capacity (lower right) have a place in this framework as well. *Biocultural* is, therefore, a term that acknowledges that the individuals we are today is the result of our unique combination of exposures to influences as varying as genes, nutrients, and cultural expectations. It is a holistic perspective that considers the opportunities and constraints presented by our biological and cultural environments and how we respond, or adapt, to them.[1]

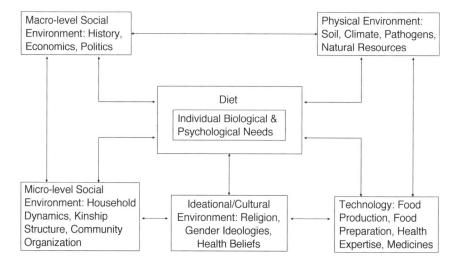

FIGURE 2.1
A biocultural, ecological model of nutrition (adapted from Jerome et al. 1980; Young and Pelto 2006).

Now you have some sense of what biocultural means, but to really understand it, it is helpful to delve into the signature characteristics of biocultural work. There are six. Biocultural research focuses on adaptation. It is both *holistic* and therefore necessarily *multidisciplinary*. Similar to other life sciences, it distinguishes across *levels of analysis*, uses the *scientific method*, and is *evidence-based*. Each of these features is discussed in turn, below.

Adaptation and Fitness

Attention to the adaptive process—how humans cope and adjust to meet material needs in response to ecological challenges—is fundamental to research in anthropology (Pelto et al. 2000) and any biocultural endeavor. Anthropologists typically distinguish three levels of adaptation (Young and Pelto 2006):

1. Genetic adaptation, e.g., the proliferation of the sickle-cell trait which is protective against malaria

2. Physiological adaptation, e.g., decreased basal metabolic rate during periods of starvation and expanded lung capacity when living at high altitudes
3. Sociocultural adaptation, e.g., the soaking of corn in an alkaline solution prior to cooking it, which frees up otherwise unavailable niacin (Katz et al. 1975)

Biocultural research tends to focus on the latter two types. It recognizes that the influence of each of the domains in figure 2.1 is not unidirectional; the human is acted upon, but is also an actor. There is room for individual choice, and thus the bidirectional arrows between each of these realms.

Much biocultural research attempts to measure if practices are beneficial to health and well-being, or not. The measurement of health is complex and has been variously quantified by frequency of illness, life expectancy, quality of life, and number of surviving offspring, among other measures. In biocultural analyses, the terms **adaptive** and *nonadaptive* are used to characterize behaviors based on their contribution to the health of an individual. *Fitness* is another metric of the adaptiveness of a behavior and is a measure of the capability of an individual to reproduce.

The fact that geophagy is widespread in the animal kingdom (cf. chapter 1) suggests there is likely some adaptive benefit. As one famous ethologist put it, unlike humans, "animals aren't messed up by culture." We can count on wild animals to behave in ways that improve the chance of survival for themselves and their offspring, at least with greater regularity than modern humans do.

Holistic

With so many relevant domains (cf. fig. 2.1), a biocultural approach is necessarily holistic, i.e., it assumes a phenomenon cannot be understood outside of the context of its physical, biological, historical, social, economic, (etc.) properties. Translating this holism to the study of pica, facts that may initially seem tangential become relevant to the etiology of pica. For example, the use of **terra sigillata** in ancient pharmacopeia (chapter 3) suggests that a number of pica substances may have detoxifying biological consequences worth exploring (chapter 9). By understanding the condemnation rained upon those who engage in pica (chapter 6), the concealment of pica becomes understandable, and techniques for collecting more accurate data become apparent (this chapter). By appreciating the special significance of clays during pregnancy (chapters 1, 4, and 6), we can focus on potential nutritional and immunological functions of pica (chapters 8 and 9). And so forth.

But such a broad perspective is easier than it sounds. It means you technically need to look at everything related to pica, which in this case meant acquiring and reading more than 3,100 references on pica (and instilling dread into the hearts of librarians across continents in the process). But as Goethe put it, "he who cannot draw on three thousand years is living hand to mouth." The many types of data that I have assimilated have their place in the testing of pica hypotheses, as you'll see in the rest of this book.[2] Without this breadth of literature, I could not present such a comprehensive description of pica.

Multidisciplinary

There is no one correct field to study pica; it takes a range of expertise to put all the hypotheses together, to identify the correct techniques for testing them, to gather appropriate data to test them, and to analyze the resulting data. However, a common shortcoming in pica research is that scientists have typically evaluated pica solely within the realm of their own discipline; nutritionists wonder if earth supplies iron, parasitologists evaluate if it spreads **geohelminths**, and geologists describe the characteristics of the soil eaten (Young et al. 2008). In fact, this lack of multidisciplinarity is one reason why pica is not better understood by now; overly narrow definitions of pica have not permitted a multidisciplinary study.[3]

Certainly, it is difficult to be aware of the ways in which pica may affect the body that fall outside of one's own discipline. To study pica properly, one needs, at the minimum, cursory familiarity with human behavior, digestion, parasitology, soil science, and epidemiology. Besides some knowledge of these fields, it's also necessary to be able to explain and translate between them for collaborators and audiences with different backgrounds. This can be a lot to ask in these days of academic sub-sub-sub-specializations. But assembling knowledge across fields can promote major advances in scientific understanding. Even U.S. government agencies have recognized that "substantial improvements in public health can be achieved as a result of increased collaboration between the earth science and public health communities" (National Research Council and Institute of Medicine 2007:141).

Romer and colleagues (1976:276) wrote that "medicine has not made any claim on geophagy, and ethnology does not take into account the chemical and pharmaceutical literature at all." Fortunately, research on pica *is* becoming more multidisciplinary. The work that anthropologist Dr. P. Wenzel Geissler did on geophagy, anemia, and geohelminth infections with colleagues from parasitology and nutrition (Aagaard-Hansen and Ouma 2002) is a great testament to the power of a multidisciplinary approach. Dr. James Gilardi, an ecologist, has successfully tested a range of hypotheses about the function of geophagy among Amazonian parrots by using methodologies from toxicology, nutrition, and mineralogy (1999). The work of Drs. Tim Johns and Martin Duquette on the function of human geophagy has been so successful in part because of their decision to test hypotheses from multiple disciplines using a range of techniques (e.g., 1991a). Similarly, without the number of cross-disciplinary collaborations with colleagues in anthropology, behavioral ecology, classical studies, food science, nutrition, parasitology, public health, and soil science, my work on pica would not be nearly as rich.

Levels of Analysis

Many a tussle has broken out among biologists as they answer questions about why organism X exhibits trait Y. The problem usually stems from a misunderstanding of levels of analysis. We have Nikolaas Tinbergen, a Dutch ornithologist and Nobel laureate, to thank for identifying the four types of questions, or levels of analysis, that can be applied to the study of a trait. Proper application of these questions can avoid much academic friction and, more importantly, further our understanding of pica. In **Tinbergen's Four Questions**, two questions deal with behavior at the level of the individual—"proximate explanations"—and two deal with the evolution of a species—"ultimate explanations."[4]

Proximate questions pertain to:

Causation (mechanisms): What are the stimuli that elicit the response, and how have recent experiences modified that behavior? For pica, this could mean eliciting the impetus for eating non-food substances, e.g., visual, olfactory, or cultural cues.

Development (ontogeny): How does the behavior change with age? For pica, this means identifying how pica fluctuates during childhood, adulthood, pregnancy, and in old age.

Ultimate questions pertain to:

Evolutionary origins (phylogeny): How does the behavior compare with similar traits in related species? Do other species engage in pica? Which ones, and how is their diet, metabolism, disease exposure similar or different from *Homo sapiens*?

Functional consequences: How does this behavior impact the animal's chances of survival and reproduction? Does pica cause people to be sicker than those who do not engage in it? Does it offer an adaptive advantage?

The levels of analysis make room for different types of answers to be possible. That is, each question can be applied to the same trait and yield a different, but still correct, answer. Dr. Paul Sherman illustrated this poetically in a discussion of the clitoris and its function(s) (Sherman 1988, 1989). Correctly identifying the stimuli that elicits an orgasm does not make the study of the consequences of orgasm on the fitness of the species any more or less right. Similarly, identifying *how* a person "knows" to eat chalk is not necessary for studying the functional consequences of chalk consumption on health.

The Scientific Method

The scientific method is a powerful approach to understanding our world. For those of you who are less familiar with falsifiable science, the scientific method is simply a way of making sure an observable phenomenon is really the result of what a scientist says it is. Fortunately, it is very straightforward.

First you make a hypothesis, a statement that can be falsified: X is caused by Y. Based on this statement, you make predictions, or describe different scenarios under which if X was true, Y would be true, and vice versa. You then collect data in the form of observations and experiments, and see how your predictions stand up against what you observe. If the data indicate that the hypothesis is false, you revise it to reflect your most recent observations, and the cycle begins again. Chapters 7, 8, and 9 are organized around such hypotheses and predictions.

Studying variations in practice across time (evolution, individual maturation), space (climate, geography), and species is integral to the biocultural approach. Such comparisons give a sense of the conditions (climactic, dietary, etc.) that are conducive to pica. These, in turn, make it possible to develop better thought-out hypotheses than are otherwise possible based on single observations.

As we move forward with our hypothesis testing, we must, of course, bear in mind the possibility that there may be multiple etiologies of the picas. For example, pagophagy may well be motivated by an entirely different phenomenon than geophagy. It's also possible that non-food consumption functions differently in different species; the metabolic and ecological challenges that face herbivores are very different than those that face carnivores or omnivores.

Evidence-based Analyses

In order to use the scientific method, you need data: And while most data are useful, not all data are created equal. Levels of certainty about the phenomenon under scrutiny increase as the quality of your data improves. *Anecdotes*, or case studies, based on just one observation are the weakest type of data.

Observations of *associations* in larger groups are a rung higher on the ladder of data quality. But association should never be confused with causation, even though it often is. In the United States, pregnancy is associated with eating ice cream and pickles, but thankfully, ice cream and pickles have never *caused* pregnancy.

Longitudinal data, data based on observations over time, are better yet. With such information you can demonstrate chronology, e.g., that pica came before (or after) **anemia**. While longitudinal data increase the plausibility of a hypothesized relationship, they are frequently not enough to prove beyond doubt that your hypothesis holds true.

Experimental data show greater rigor for two main reasons. They can show dose response, e.g., that the more earth you eat the more anemic you become. Most importantly, good experiments control for what are known as **confounders**, phenomena that affect both the cause and the effect under study. Pregnancy is a good example of a confounder in the pica–anemia–pregnancy love triangle. Pregnancy is strongly associated with pica, and pregnancy also causes anemia (more on this in chapter 8).

The most convincing data are those which can demonstrate the *mechanism* by which effect Y is manifested. Demonstrating how pica substances could cause anemia, for example, would lend support to the causal arrow going from pica to anemia. Mechanistic evidence is the type of data that really seals the deal.

In this book you will encounter all of these types of data, although there are more anecdotes and associations than rigorous experimental data. Sophisticated scientific study of pica is really only beginning. Such a range of data quality isn't a bad thing; indeed biocultural research depends on a range of types of evidence. It was an anecdotal remark that brought pica to my attention, and ethnographic data from Pemba that made me wonder if pica wasn't perhaps worth further investigation. The repeated associations between pregnancy, anemia, and pica suggested the importance of the study and indicated which hypotheses were the most promising.[5] Experimental evidence will be presented in later chapters to examine the viability of the hypotheses. In short, science cannot make progress with mere conjecture; hypothesis testing requires data, and many types of it. As you read, you will notice that the quality of the data to test pica hypotheses is frequently low. The field of pica is ready for more experimental data.

Pica Data in This Book

Although I rely on many types of data in this book (cf. note 2), there are two sources to which I refer at length. The first is the Pica Literature Database; the second is an epidemiological study among pregnant Pemban women.

The Pica Literature Database

Once the lay of the pica land is revealed through holistic endeavors, comparisons across time, space, and species become easier. Drs. Paul Sherman, Julius Lucks, Gretel Pelto, and I developed the Pica Literature Database in order to do just this. Our database includes every obtainable, culture-level report of pica.[6] To date, we have identified 472 such publications. Among these 472 publications, there are 361 distinct cultural reports of geophagy from all over the world. Because information on geophagy spans two thousand years and includes reports from ethnographers, colonial explorers, government officials, missionaries, medical doctors, nurses, nutritionists, and journalists, the quality and detail of observations vary widely. Some reports of geophagy are lengthy (more than twenty pages) and describe in detail which individuals practice geophagy, when in their lifetimes they do so, sources and preparation of soil, costs, etc. Other reports are no more than brief mentions, e.g., a single phrase in a 417-page ethnographic study. This uneven data mean that for each phenomenon we examine, such as the physical characteristics of earth or the timing of geophagy onset, we have widely fluctuating denominators.

Besides the irregular quality of the descriptions of pica, this database also encounters limitations in textual evidence. We know that pica is much older than the written word and likely dates back to *Homo habilis* (Clark 2001), but available archaeological data are incommensurate with the probable frequency of the behavior. Another limitation is that many of the references come from European authors who were frequently judgmental of the populations they described. Although derogatory explanations are part of the database, such attitudes may have caused biased reporting.

For each article, we extracted available information on all of the following variables: year of observation, geographic location, climate, non-food materials consumed (appearance, source, preparation), life stage of the consumer (child, adolescent, pregnant, etc.), and any associations with physiological conditions, such as gastrointestinal distress, anemia, and hunger. If several reports were made about earth eaten by the same group of people or in the same area within a ten-year span, but by different authors, these were combined into one cultural report.

We grouped geophagy by seven life stages.[7] Data on exact proportions of populations or subpopulations that engaged in geophagy were rarely given in the reports we compiled. Rather, qualitative terms like "some," "all," "frequently," and "rarely" were used instead. In an attempt to quantify these descriptive terms, we constructed a scoring system from 0 to 5 (table 2.1) based on that of Wiley and Katz (1998). Geophagy scores were then determined by averaging across the descriptions of geophagy frequency by life stage.

I will be referring to the Pica Literature Database throughout the following chapters, so it will be helpful to understand the geophagy score: the

TABLE 2.1
Geophagy Scoring System Used in the Operationalization of Geophagy Frequency

Score	Term Associated
0	Never
1	Rarely, few
2	Sometimes, occasionally
3	Frequently, common, habit, very common, quite general, many, endemic, widely, often
4	Usually, typically
5	Always

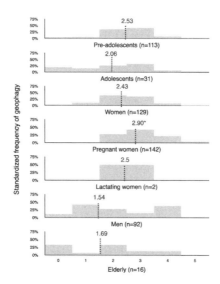

FIGURE 2.2
Standardized geophagy frequencies and mean geophagy score (vertical dotted line) by life stage (based on culture-level reports of geophagy in the Pica Literature Database).

lower the number, the less frequent the geophagy. Based on figure 2.2, in which geophagy score is plotted by life stage, it becomes clear that pregnant women have the highest geophagy score (2.90), followed by preadolescents (2.53). Men (1.54) and the elderly (1.69) have the lowest geophagy scores.

Epidemiological Study Among Pregnant Pembans

The *Mama na Afya*, or Mothers and Health study, was a clinical trial whose objective was to study two different medicine and micronutrient regimens to reduce severe anemia during pregnancy.[8] This study made it possible to collect data on biological indices and behavioral patterns associated with pica, as well as to examine the biochemical properties of pica substances themselves.

It was conducted in 2004 and 2005 among 2,368 pregnant Pembans who were recruited from public antenatal health clinics at their first antenatal visit, which in Pemba happens around the sixth month of pregnancy. Because nearly 98% of Pemban women attend a public antenatal clinic at some point during pregnancy, this sample is likely representative of the obstetric population.

Most women enrolled in the study had three visits with study staff; some had more if they were involved in a follow-up study. In the course of the study, the growth of the fetus was measured, blood samples were taken to test iron and malaria status, and in a subsample of women a stool sample was collected to test for geohelminth infection.

Women were also asked about health-related behaviors, including pica. Before the study began, a list of pica substances most commonly consumed on Pemba was generated using a free listing technique. Pembans were asked, "Which substances do you like to eat that are not normal food?" This longer list consisted of unripe mango, husked but uncooked rice, four types of earth, and large quantities of ice, charcoal, ash, chalk, whitewash, baby powder, and powdered shell. Pica behaviors were asked about at numerous time points: prior to current pregnancy; at any time during the current pregnancy; at the time of that visit; and two weeks after delivery. Information on current pica practices was available for all but one of the 2,368 women enrolled, and on postpartum pica practices for 67% of the sample. In order to obtain prospective data on pica behaviors in a non-pregnant population, 568 male and female household members of a subsample of study participants were also surveyed.

Additionally, in-depth interviews about pica were conducted with a purposive sample of men and women who had professed pica behavior (n = 53). The in-depth interviews lasted from 30 to 75 minutes and covered topics including sample identification, collection, storage, and preparation as well as the attractiveness of various qualities, e.g., color, texture, flavor. After the interview, a Pemban fieldworker and/or I accompanied participants to the source of the pica substance if they were still engaging in pica. The consumer then collected precise amounts of the materials he or she consumed, as well as a large amount for subsequent analysis.

In this chapter, I have described the biocultural perspective, one that considers both physiological and social facets of behavior and health. Such a perspective is not an easy one because it takes a holistic approach that requires familiarity with content and methodologies from multiple disciplines. The biocultural perspective also requires scientific rigor: for distinction across different types of *why* questions, for hypotheses development, and for their testing by applying the scientific method to a variety of types of data.

Although a biocultural approach is not straightforward, its many fruits make it a worthwhile endeavor. Not only does it permit a schema for organizing a fascinating, but messy, array of information, it helps pica to be regarded with scientific objectivity rather than emotional judgments, so that the true adaptive value of pica can come to light.

CHAPTER THREE

Medicine You Can Walk On

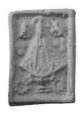 NOT ALL GEOPHAGY is pica. Inadvertently swallowing a clod of dirt in your freshly picked arugula or politely smacking your lips on your son's mud pie are indeed geophagy, but pica are they not. You'll recall from chapter 1 that one component of the definition of pica is that it involves strong cravings. Thus, because neither of these instances includes a *desire* for earth, they would not be considered pica, although they are both geophagy.

This chapter is about non-pica geophagy in the field of medicine. How is that germane to a book about pica? Most importantly, understanding the healing powers with which pica substances have long been imbued provides clues to the function of pica. As an added bonus, some fascinating details about the role of religion and science in mundane modern pharmaceuticals are unveiled. Because all earths used in medicine are clay-rich, I shall begin by discussing a few of the physical and chemical features of **clay**.

The Amazing Properties of Clays

Although they may seem lackluster, clays are actually capable of dynamic and astounding feats. They are also very complex; many scientists have

dedicated their entire lives to their study. What follows is a cursory introduction to what clays are and how they interact with their environments.
Both pieces of information are critical for discussions throughout the rest
of the book.

What Is a Clay?

Soil is made up of both organic and inorganic constituents. The part where
most microbial activity happens is in the **humus,** the rich, dark brown stuff
mostly made of decayed organic matter. (You'll recall from chapter 1 that
geophagists stay away from humus-rich soil.) The inorganic components
are essentially the product of the parent rock(s) from which the soil derives.
They may closely resemble the boulder from which they eroded, or they
may be greatly altered by weathering, which causes the rock to decompose
into various particle sizes. In descending size order, these are medium to
coarse sand (0.2–2 mm), fine sand (0.02–0.20 mm), silt (0.002–0.02 mm,
still visible to the naked eye), and clay (<0.002 mm, impossible to see an
individual particle). Here's an indication of the magnitude of size differences. If you drop a particle of course sand in water, it will fall about 10 cm
in 1 second. A particle of silt will fall 10 cm in about 5 minutes. A particle
of clay will take 860 years to fall the same 10 cm (Logan 1995:116). As
we shall see, this very small particle size makes clays extremely useful in a
range of applications.

There are several types of clay minerals (Loveland et al. 1989; Millot
1979: see also table 3.1). Scientists use the term **clay minerals** to refer to
groups of clays with similar layer structures. Clay minerals are all phyllo-
silicates, a category of silicate minerals made up of parallel sheets, usually
of an aluminosilicate ("phyllo" means sheet). The term *clay* is used to refer
to materials that consist largely of different sorts of clay minerals (Millot
1979).

Clays, the smallest particles in rocks, are fascinating for many reasons,
including their physical structure. If you look at granite, say, on a fancy
kitchen countertop, you can easily see its crystalline structure. Clays, too,
have similar crystalline structures, only theirs are microscopic (Millot
1979). Geochemist Dr. Lynda Williams, whose work on medicinal clays
is discussed at the end of this chapter, describes clay crystal structures by
way of an analogy to a peanut butter and jelly sandwich (Coulombe 2007).
The slices of bread in the clay structure are extremely thin layers of flat
aluminosilicate sheets that are negatively charged. These negative surfaces

TABLE 3.1
Characteristics of the Clay Mineral Groups

Clay Mineral Group	Example of Clay	CEC* (mEq/100g)
Mica	Illite	20–40
Kaolin	Kaolinite, halloysite	2–10
Palygorskite	Fuller's earth	8–22
(formerly known as attapulgite)		
Smectite	Montmorillonite,	80–175
formerly known as montmorillonite)	saponite	

* Cation exchange capacity
Note: Adapted from (Loveland et al. 1989; Millot 1979).

attract positively charged atoms, called **cations**. Examples of cations include Fe^{3+}, Fe^{2+}, Mg^{2+}, and K^+. Cations may be thought of as the peanut butter on the bread. Continuing the analogy, the jelly is composed of organic compounds that are also sometimes adsorbed[1] between the silicate layers.

Clays have the ability to adsorb a wide variety of molecules, especially when they are dispersed in water. A measure of how readily a substance can exchange adsorbed cations—those positively charged molecules stuck to the "bread"—with cations in a surrounding solution is called the **cation exchange capacity** (**CEC**). If the cation exchange capacity is low, a clay mineral is less likely to form an insoluble complex with cations. If the cation exchange capacity is high, cations are likely to become bound tightly to the substance and thus be unavailable to be metabolized. Cation exchange capacity varies enormously, from about 2mEq/100g in kaolinite to approximately 150mEq/100g in some smectites. The likelihood of cation exchange also depends on the strength of charge of the cations in solution. The stronger the charge of the cation already bound to the "bread," the less likely it will be replaced by another cation. For example, Fe^{3+} cannot ordinarily be replaced by Fe^{2+}.

In addition to the binding capacity it makes possible, such a crystal structure is also responsible for clays' high surface-to-volume ratios. There is only a small amount of accessible interior space when the parent minerals are still part of a rock, but as they weather into small clay particles, the surface area greatly increases. For some perspective, one gram of clay can have a surface area larger than a football field (Logan 1995:125).

Industrial Uses of Clay

There are many industrial uses of clay, all of which are based on its extraordinary binding capacity. Fuller's earth, also known as calcium montmorillonite, was used for centuries to absorb lanolin, oils, and other greasy impurities in wools (Robertson 1986). Today, most landfills include a layer of clay to prevent contamination of the groundwater by the sludge that oozes out of our trash. In fact, clay liners are used in all kinds of waste management contraptions, including lagoons and ponds built to contain liquid wastes and berms to contain spills. Clays are used to clean up massive oil spills and to isolate radioactive waste. The clay in kitty litter helps to absorb the pungent smell of Felix's business. And clays are used to filter vegetable oils, remove heavy metals from wastewater, and purify the air we breathe. Think, too, of the mud masks applied to draw out impurities that would otherwise mar our pretty faces, and the mud baths, considered therapeutic for their beautifying and cleansing powers.[2] In short, clays are excellent at removing unwanted molecules.

The small particle size of clays also makes them useful in the paper industry. In fact, they function similarly to starches in paper production (more on this under "Starch" in ch. 9, p. 126). Clays are used to smooth out paper and cardboard by filling in the crevices around the wood pulp. Clays are also used to coat paper, to prevent the bleeding of ink (Millot 1979).

When it is dusted on surfaces, the fine powderiness of clay makes it an effective barrier against insects, too. How? As insects land on clay-dusted surfaces, the clay works its way into the waxy coating of their bodies; it is microscopically abrasive. Eventually, these cuts and scratches cause insects to shrivel and die. It's a pest-control strategy that is gaining popularity, for there are a number of advantages: it's not a poison; it doesn't lose potency over time; and it is not harmful to most larger animals.[3] In short, this myriad of uses of clays means you can probably find them in every room of your house, from garage to bathroom.

Early Pharmacopeia

The Rise and Fall of Terra Sigillata

Saltwater taffy–sized hunks of clay from a tiny Greek island were once literally worth their weight in gold (fig. 3.1). This clay was called **terra sigillata**, which means "stamped earth" (*sigillum*, Latin for "seal"). The "stamp" refers

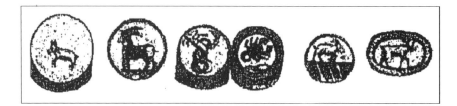

FIGURE 3.1
Earliest examples of terra sigillata, when goats were prominent on the seal (Thompson 1914).

to a mark of quality or origin pressed into the clay, much like the signet rings that kings and queens pressed into melted wax to seal their royal missives.[4]

Terra sigillata was so valuable because of its healing properties, as espoused by the medical literature of the time. Admittedly, in the first century C.E. there was not a wide variety of medical literature to choose from. In the Roman Empire, there was Pliny's *Naturalis Historia* (Pliny/Rackham 1952) and in Greece, Dioscorides' *De Materia Medica* (Dioscorides et al. 1934); both discussed the medicinal uses of terra sigillata.[5] (Appendix A may help you to contextualize the historical events described here.)

Pliny wrote about terra sigillata in several sections: how it could be used as an antidote to swallowed poisons and snakebites, as a treatment for dysentery, and to reduce inflammation around the eyes (Pliny/Rackham 1952). Of terra sigillata, Dioscorides wrote:

> But it hath an eminent faculty of antidot against deadly poisons when drank with wine, & being taken before, it constrains to vomit up poisons. It is good also against ye strokes & it is good for ye bitings of venemous poison-outcasting beasts. It is mixed also with Antidotes. And some also use it for expiations. And it is good also for dysenteries. (Bk. 5, ch. 113)

But what, exactly, was this mysterious terra sigillata? First-century readers could not know for another one hundred years, until 167 C.E., when the great physician Galen visited the Greek island of Lemnos, the source of terra sigallata. His visit was the world's first eyewitness account of its collection (Tozer 1890).[6] He described the solemn production of terra sigillata with great detail:

> The priestess collects this, to the accompaniment of some local ceremony, no animals being sacrificed, but wheat and barley being given back to

the land in exchange. She then takes it to the city, mixes it with water so as to make moist mud, shakes this violently and then allows it to stand. Thereafter she removes first the superficial water, and next the greasy part of the earth below this, leaving only the stony and sandy part at the bottom, which is useless. She now dries the greasy mud until it reaches the consistency of soft wax. Of this she takes small portions and imprints upon them the seal of Artemis, namely the goat, then again she dries these in the shade till they are absolutely free from moisture. (Cited in Brock 1929:194)

Galen subscribed wholeheartedly to the medicinal properties of these seals; indeed, he took 20,000 tablets with him back to Rome.

Fueled by the praises of these esteemed physicians, the popularity and price of terra sigillata increased over the next centuries until they were "considered equivalent with gold" (Thompson 1914:440). By then, they were used by physicians, healers, and midwives throughout Europe to treat smallpox, dysentery, and pestilential (epidemic-causing) diseases (Forestus/ Burri 1982 [1557]; Mérat and de Lens 1834; Salmon 1691). Sometimes it was used by itself and other times as part of a concoction of cryptic ingredients like treacle of Andromicus and Hungary powder. In addition to treating illnesses, it was also used preventatively: royalty swallowed a tablet with their meals as a safeguard against being poisoned (Thorndike 1923). By the end of the sixteenth century, terra sigillata was in such great demand that ambassadors "were accustomed to take supplies of it with them to present to distinguished men" (Thompson 1914:440).

In fact, Lemnian earth had become so desired and so costly that it was frequently counterfeited and "almost every country in Europe strove to find within its boundaries a source of supply of so valuable and profitable a commodity" (Thompson 1914:435). Eventually, other earths did gain repute, including those from Silesia, Poland (called Terra sigillata Strigoniensis), Samos, Greece (Terra sigillata Samia), Sicily (Terra sigillata Sicula), and Jerusalem (Terra sigillata Hierosolymitanae, rhymes with Jerusalemitan) (Mérat and de Lens 1834). And just like in Lemnos, earths from these places had their own special seals (Dannenfeldt 1984). Terra sigillata was soon no longer synonymous with the sealed earth tablets from Lemnos, but rather with a whole variety of earths (Dannenfeldt 1984).

This value and fame incited a multitude of travelers to visit Lemnos.[7] Pierre Belon, a French naturalist, was one such visitor and provided one of the most informative accounts of the extraction of the earth for terra sigillata (Belon 1588). His sixteenth-century description reflected the

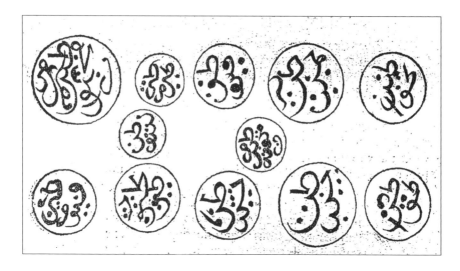

FIGURE 3.2
Lemnian terra sigillata from the time of Turkish occupation (Belon 1588).

changes in religion, control of natural resources, and political power wrought by the many wars between Turkey and Greece. For example, by the sixteenth century, Hellenic priestesses had been replaced by male Christian priests and monks[8] and the digging only happened once a year, before sunrise on August 6. Prior to the removal of earth, Christian priests held a mass in a little chapel that had been built at the foot of the hill. Muslim religious authorities, called *khodjas*, also participated in the ceremony by sacrificing a lamb. The mass was well attended, with more than 3,000 in the crowd; even the Ottoman governor, who was Muslim, was there.

The priests presided over the collection of earth, and it took fifty or sixty diggers to reach the depth where the holy earth was found; it was no longer the solitary endeavor of a priestess. Up to seven mule loads of earth were taken, most of which was sent to Constantinople, the then capital of the Ottoman empire. Another change since Galen's visit was that the seal pressed into the clay pieces was no longer a goat; after the Turkish Muslim occupation of Lemnos, this idolatry was replaced with the script *tyn mahktoum* (Mérat and de Lens 1834), meaning hidden, concealed, and/or secret mud (fig. 3.2).

We know from the English scholar, Henry Tozer, that by 1890, interest in the ceremony was on the decline:

[It] is evident from the neglect into which it has lately fallen, that ere long it will be a thing of the past. For several years the Turkish governor has ceased to attend, and, following his example, first the *khodjas* and then the priests absented themselves, and no lamb is now sacrificed. Last year only twelve persons were present. Though the tablets were to be bought in chemists' shops in Kastro at the time of Conze's visit to the island in 1858, I enquired in vain for them; and neither the existing governor, nor any persons of the younger generation, had heard of this remedy. In the eastern parts of Lemnos, however, it is still in use for fevers and some other disorders, for the women possess nuts of it, which they string like the beads of a rosary; these they grate in case of illness, and take a tea-spoonful of the powder in water. Not long ago the proprietor of the hill-side applied for leave to plough over the spot and sow it with corn; and though for the time this was not allowed by the government, yet, when the annual celebration has come to an end, the prohibition will safely be ignored, and from that time forward the locality itself will be forgotten. (Tozer 1890:265–66)

Lemnian Earth Today

Is Lemnian terra sigillata still obtainable? To answer this question, es-teemed food geographer Professor Louis Grivetti at the University of Cali-fornia, Davis, went to Lemnos on a quest similar to Galen's. On August 6, 1984, he hired a taxi and driver, Tsokhas, to bring him to Kotsinos (Greek: Κότσινος), the alleged site of the holy earth. If Grivetti's efforts sound quix-otic, Tsokhas was, as you'll see, his Sancho.

After the airport, the road to Kotsinos was rough. . . . The road wors-ened and we reached the sea. There is Kotsinos, Tsokhas said—my first view. This view was one of semi-shock; Kotsinos consisted of 3–5 houses, a whitewashed church on a mound (archaeological mound?) and the bronze statue of Morula [heroine of Lemnos]. But where were the pil-grims? Where were the hundreds coming from all over the island to cel-ebrate the Iasus Soteros on August 6th? I expected busloads, cars, carts, people walking, milling about, the air of a traditional feast celebration. There was not a sound—or any activity!

Tsokhas drove into "town" past a taverna and parked. One fisherman was visible on the breakwater; two men were sitting in front of the café. We greeted them, and spoke to the owner, a woman. . . . Yes, the site for digging the clay was nearby along the southwestern hillside (as the guidebooks said)—but each asked why we wanted to go there? No one goes there; no one digs the clay—that was in the time only of the Turkish Sultans. No priest—in their lifetime of memory—had ever blessed the ground; but they used to do so in the time of the Sultans. The priest would go before dawn on one day of the year—not August 6th—and bless the ground, and the clay would "come forth from the ground like toothpaste." It would be collected, and given to people, especially used by the Turks to test for poison. . . .

With great anticipation we (at least I, for Tsokhas was not looking forward to the next stage) drove to the southwest and parked. We walked through a recently harvested wheat field and hailed a shepherd (and his two dogs) who welcomed us. Yes, the clay site was on the hill, just around the eastern spur, midway up the slope. We should go there, find another person, and ask permission to dig. I was really excited; the link with past and present was flowing and I could sense this wonderful feeling of anticipation.

The total site was covered with thistle, star thorn, and other weeds. Simple digging was all gravel and loose rock! No fine clay sediment! I was very disappointed. Tsokhas, hoe in hand, sat on the vertical rock at the east end. I climbed to the crest of the hill and looked down on the scene. A strange "V" trench snaked below me. The two stones were clearly at the northeast end of a rectangular depression; it looked like a church foundation. Two donkeys grazed beyond the stones; we had not seen them earlier. Below me to the north was Kotsinos, the church, and ugly Morula gazing seaward! Legends and hopes die hard; it was time to leave. (Grivetti, unpublished fieldnotes)

The poor professor took the disappointment rather hard, as reflected by his poem, "Old Dreams Die Hard," penned that very day.

Old dreams die hard.
When truth reveals a different vision of the past,
Embellished myth that cannot last,
Old dreams die hard.

Old dreams die hard.
The search for truth is endless and must ever stand,
Upsetting theories built on sand,
Old dreams die hard.

Grivetti's discovery of a whole lot of nothing in the way of terra sigillata on Lemnos has since been confirmed by a 1992 visit by a *Financial Times* journalist (Spence 1993) and a visit by a scholar, Rudolph Reinbacher, in 2000 (2002). During Reinbacher's visit, he did, however, get a sample of clay-based antidiarrheal medicine from his taxi driver's mother.[9] Ironically, the local pharmacist decried it, and recommended a far more expensive preparation: Kaopectate.

Beyond Europe

Europe was not the only place where clay was sought after as medicine. Earth has long had a place in the Chinese pharmacopeia. Ch'en Nan, a Taoist *Xian* (a person who transcends mortality) born in the early 1200s, had the power of curing diseases with medicine made of earth kneaded with charmed water. Although he was most famous for floating across a river standing on his hat, the healing properties of this medicine earned him the nickname "Mud-pill Ch'en" (Yetts 1919).

The sixteenth-century Chinese physician Li Shizhen listed pharmacological uses for sixty-one clays, muds, and other earths in the most complete and comprehensive medical book on the history of traditional Chinese medicine, *Bencao Gangmu*. The earths he listed could treat conditions from malnutrition to infection to diarrhea. Unfortunately, many are described too obtusely to identify today, e.g., "soil underneath the shoe," "soil from the northwest of China." Healing earth also made its way into a French missionary's encyclopedic survey of everything Chinese, described as "a certain soft Stone or Mineral, call'd Hiung hoang, of which they make Vessels; and the Physicians esteem it as a sovereign Remedy against all sorts of Poison, malignant Fevers, and contagious Heats in the Dog-Days" (Du Halde 1741:226–27).

In fact, around the world, a number of earths found their way among the cinnabar, frankincense, unicorn horns, and dried newts on physicians' shelves. In parts of the world that valued the written word, the many recommended uses of earth are well documented. Clays show up in inventories of materia medica in Sumeria (Ebers 1889), India (Chopra 1933; Dutt et al. 1980; Jee 1896), the Middle East (Budge 1913; Guiges 1905; Ibn el-Beithar and Leclerc 1877; Mohaghegh 1976), and South America (Cobo and de la Espada 1890).

In places where the written word was less central, proof that earths have been used to treat a variety of maladies comes from reports by outsiders. Some were important during fertility and birth. For example, clay was thought to facilitate a quick delivery and expulsion of afterbirth in Mongolia (Pallas 1776), and a handful of fine clay in wine was drunk to avoid a spontaneous abortion in the Canary Islands (de Hoyos Sáinz and de Hoyos Sancho 1947). Most of the documented uses, however, were related to the treatment of gastrointestinal ills. In the Congo, red clay was used to quell diarrhea (Costermans 1895); Australian aborigines (Roth and Etheridge 1897) and Native Americans in the Great Lakes region (Kinietz and Raudot 1965) used clay pills for the same purpose. In the Philippines, clay was used to treat cholera and dysentery (Cole and Gale 1922) and in Siberia, bright yellow chalky earth called *stone butter* was used to treat cholera (Muller 1722).

Modern Medicine

It may come as a surprise, but earth remains in our modern pharmacopeia, although the snazzy packaging does much to disguise the active ingredients. As described below, it is used both internally and topically.

Clays have been scientifically validated as effective treatments for diarrhea (more on this is chapter 9). In fact, you may have already swigged some clay, albeit in far more industrialized wrapping than old Mud Pill Ch'en offered his ailing clientele. Kaopectate™, the largest-selling over-the-counter medicine for nausea and diarrhea in the United States, gets its name from the original active ingredient—kaolin, one type of clay.[10] However, clay is no longer the active ingredient due to formulation changes in the 1990s, and as such, Kaopectate is a misnomer.[11]

Other clays, however, do remain in current medical use. Smectite (another type of clay) is the active ingredient in a preparation that quells heartburn and diarrhea called Smecta™, and is used quite regularly to treat gastrointestinal problems in Europe, Asia, and Africa.[12] Clinical studies on smectite and diarrhea in children have demonstrated that smectite administered with oral rehydration solution (an electrolyte mixture that prevents dehydration) shortens the course of diarrhea by an entire day, compared to just oral rehydration solution by itself (Szajewska et al. 2006).

The second major application of clays in modern medicine is external, for wound healing. This use is also very old. Galen reports that clay promoted the closure of wounds, including the bite of a mad dog; Pliny mentions it as a remedy for ulcers in the humid parts of the body such as the mouth or anus. The popularity of topically administered clays has waxed and waned over the centuries, but interest in healing properties of clay re-surged in the late nineteenth century in both the United States (thanks to the efforts of a surgeon, Dr. Addinell Hewson), and in Germany (thanks to the efforts of Dr. Julius Stumpf) (Reinbacher 2002).[13]

Dr. Hewson's inspiration for the treatment of his patients' infected wounds with clay was a little-known invention called an Earth Closet, a kind of chamber pot that you "flushed" by dropping earth over your de-posit. He reasoned that the deodorizing power of clay made it a likely can-didate for disinfecting wounds. Indeed, it seemed to work wonders for his patients. Hewson filled a book, *Earth as a Topical Application in Surgery*, with 93 case studies and photographs of his successful non-infected ampu-tations (Hewson 1872; see also fig. 3.3).

In Germany, Dr. Stumpf's attention was called to the desiccating effects of clay when he attended the exhumation of a woman who had died shortly after giving birth. Although she had been buried for more than three years, he was astounded to see that her body was still intact, right down to where the placenta had been attached to the uterine wall. He noticed that the earth in which she had been buried was very clayey; this observation, to-gether with some reading of Pliny and Galen, caused him to hypothesize that clay might resist decomposition because it was inhospitable to bacterial growth.

Shortly after this observation, he was called to treat an old man with rank, putrid bedsores that exposed his tibia in two places. Stumpf decided that an amputation was necessary, but the old man refused. With no other recourse, he dusted what was then known as *bolus alba*, more commonly known as kaolinite, a fine, powdery white clay, on the sores. The odor was soon gone and the wounds healed shortly thereafter, obviating the amputa-tion. Stumpf proceeded to treat a number of badly infected wounds with this clay. Wounds from infected amputations, dog bites, and gory rifle ac-cidents all healed after bandaging the infected site with clay compresses.

Emboldened by this topical success, Stumpf began to explore the poten-tial for clay to heal internal problems. We can surmise that his conviction about the utility of this treatment was very strong: his first patient was his 81-year-old mother! She was vomiting violently, with severe cramps and diarrhea. He gave her clay with a little water twice an hour, and much to everyone's amazement, she had recovered by the following morning. After this success, he used clay to treat other patients with severe diarrhea and vomiting, all of whom experienced similar recuperation. When cholera broke out in Germany in 1904, Stumpf was summoned to oversee the treat-ment of those infected using white clay. His efforts were successful, and for

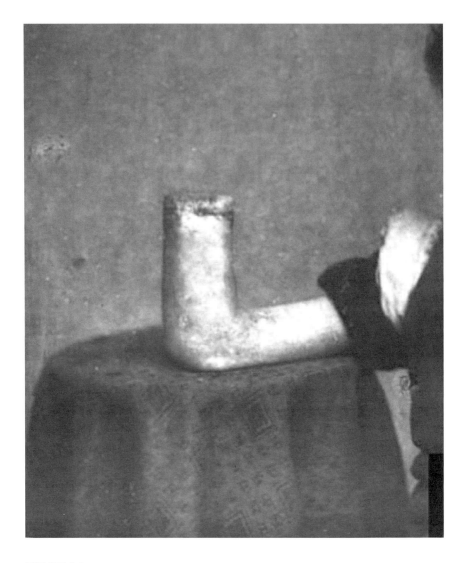

FIGURE 3.3
Dr. Addinell Hewson's infection-free handiwork (1872).

this he was decorated by several governments and received 300 free packets of bolus alba from Merck Pharmaceuticals. Another result of his medical successes is that white clay caught on in Germany. Bolus alba began to be used to treat diphtheria, gangrene, and eczema, and to prevent infections of the umbilical cord of newborn babies.

Despite these apparent successes, clays have never caught on in mainstream surgical medicine in the United States or Europe.[14] Hewson was ridiculed by his American colleagues for using "dirt" in his treatments. And just as Stumpf's work was gaining momentum, antibiotics were discovered, and these wonder drugs seemed to resolve most patients' infections.

However, now that we are facing increasing problems with antibiotic resistance, attention is once again being turned to topical uses of clay. Geochemist Dr. Lynda Williams and microbiologist Dr. Shelley Haydel at Arizona State University are studying the detoxifying properties of clays from around the world and have discovered that a handful are able to kill bacteria of major public health threats, like methicillin-resistant *Staphylococcus* infections and Buruli ulcers (a mycobacterium) (Haydel et al. 2008). It seems the scientific community's interest in the medicinal properties of clay is coming full circle.

CHAPTER FOUR

Religious Geophagy

Sacredness You Can Swallow

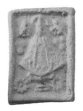 WE HAVE seen that although the extraction of terra sigillata on Lemnos occurred according to religious traditions, it was esteemed by physicians and princes neither because of the divinity of those who extracted it nor the hallowed ground from which it came. Instead, it was highly regarded because of its medicinal powers. There are, however, a number places in which earth is ingested or topically applied because of its purported religious properties. This chapter contains stories of modern-day religious geophagy from around the world, in Christianity, Islam, Hinduism, and hoodoo. It may at first seem tangential to the main storyline, since religiously prescribed geophagy is not pica. However, the healing properties frequently ascribed to earth allude to the potential curative powers of geophagy. They also help shift geophagic earth away from its lingering "dirty" connotations; in many of the examples in this chapter, earth is considered pure and holy.

Christianity

The Milk Grotto

In Bethlehem, the street heading east from Manger Square leads past the Church of the Nativity to the Milk Grotto, a cave in which Mary, Joseph, and little baby Jesus took refuge during their flight from Bethlehem and King Herod.[1] According to legend, during their respite, as Mary nursed Jesus, a drop of her milk spilled onto the cave floor. As the drop of milk touched the earth, a miracle occurred: the entire cave turned white (Canaan 1925:188; Jellingshaus 1877:50). Today this cave is known as the Grotto of the Lady Mary, or the Milk Grotto for short; in Arabic, it's Magharet Sitti Mariam.

Extraordinary properties of fertility are attributed to the soft white chunks of earth from the cave walls by people of many faiths.[2] Some women visit the shrine and ingest earth from the grotto to ensure a plentiful supply of milk for their babies. However, couples that have difficulty conceiving are the most frequent visitors. Although tablets of clay from the grotto impressed with the figure of Mary are no longer sold, humble white chunks of earth are available to all visitors. Some visitors place the small white chunks under their mattresses, others consume them on site. Brother Lawrence, whose responsibility it is to oversee the shrine for the Franciscan Custody of the Holy Land, advises on proper ingestion: "According to Catholic tradition, both the husband and wife must drink a bit of the powder mixed with milk or water for nine days and recite the prayer for the third joyful mystery of the rosary" (Sudilovsky 2007). He makes just one proviso—that the powder's mystery probably will not work on those who do not have faith. But many couples seem to have ample faith; Brother Lawrence has been told of 1,700 babies born in the last ten years due to the fertility-inducing powers of this earth. Testimonies to its powers fill the chapel:

> One picture on the wall of the Milk Grotto's chapel shows a mother from Argentina happily nursing her newborn baby. In another letter a mother from Spain wrote, "Carmen is a gift from heaven." A couple from Ireland wrote, "In thanksgiving and deep gratitude to Our Blessed Lady for our dear son Jamie." Another mother from India described how she and her husband had given up on a child after nine years of trying to conceive. Now, she wrote, after the birth of their daughter, her "whole life will be a life of thanksgiving." From Venezuela another woman wrote how after five miscarriages she gave birth to a "miracle baby, Leonardo Jose." (Sudilovsky 2007)

Esquipulas, Guatemala

Clays imbued with Christian religious significance are not unique to the Holy Land. In the thirteenth century Marco Polo described how Christians visiting St. Thomas Aquinas's tomb in India would "take a small portion of red earth, carry it into their country and give a small portion to any person sick of fever, who is presently cured" (Marco Polo et al. 1863:267). And holy earth, variously referred to as *benditos, panecitos, tierra santa,* and *pan del señor* has been documented in Catholic practices in the Americas from New Mexico to Honduras (Hunter et al. 1989).

The heart of Central American religious geophagy, however, is Esquipulas, a small town in eastern Guatemala. Each year, on January 15, throngs of pilgrims travel by foot, bus, donkey, car, and airplane to visit the Basilica, the Shrine of the Black Christ,[3] and to eat the holy earth there. Esquipulas was a holy site long before a gleaming white basilica was built there, and before Pope John Paul II proclaimed it "the spiritual center of Central America." The area was known for its health-giving earth and clear-flowing springs even before the Mayan Chorti Indians were forcibly resettled there as part of the Spanish "pacification process" in the early sixteenth century (Hunter and de Kleine 1984). Once the Chorti were resettled in present-day Esquipulas, they venerated the earth and river there.

Once they were resettled in present-day Esquipulas, the Chorti venerated the earth and river there, but the Catholic Church forbade such worship, at least until Spanish colonialists built a chapel over the sacred site in 1578. Over time, the veneration of the earth, which was initially forbidden by the Catholic Church, became manifested in geophagy[4] and assimilated into Catholic beliefs, and it remains an important activity to the throngs of pilgrims who visit Esquipulas today.

At least one million people visit Esquipulas every year and quite a few of them eat earth. In 1989, 67% of 454 surveyed adult pilgrims consumed *benditos* (Hunter et al. 1989). Men, women, and children ingest the tablets, but pregnant women are the main consumers. Benditos' miraculous properties are primarily related to fertility and birth, just as they are at the Milk Grotto; they are said to protect pregnancies, ensure safe deliveries, and counteract morning sickness.

The production of benditos is highly labor-intensive, and there are abundant parallels to the preparation of terra sigillata (cf. chapter 3). Miners, mostly men, excavate hundreds of thousands of pounds of earth from shallow caves a few miles from the Basilica (Hunter et al. 1989). They transport the clay home on donkeys, where women pound it into small pieces,

48

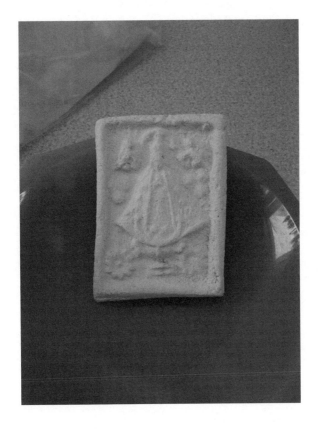

FIGURE 4.1
Bendito from Esquipulas, Guatemala, impressed with the image of the Virgin Mary and baby Jesus (In upper right). (*Photo*: S. L. Young).

crush it on a grinding stone, and finally sift it through a very fine nylon sieve. They add water to the fine powdery earth and roll out long sausage-like coils. Ceramic and wooden molds that have been dusted with clay are pressed into the long coils of dough, much like a shortbread mold. They are then sliced into squares and left in the sun to bake for a day or two (fig. 4.1). Fancier tablets are dotted with red food coloring, a symbol of the blood of Christ. Households can make tens of thousands of tablets every year.

Some families sell their benditos on tables in front of the Basilica, along with rosaries, crucifixes, and candles. Others are bought by wholesalers, who cram their pickups full of cardboard boxes of them before stopping off at the Basilica to have them blessed. Benediction happens up to six times per day at the Basilica, and there are frequently long lines of delivery

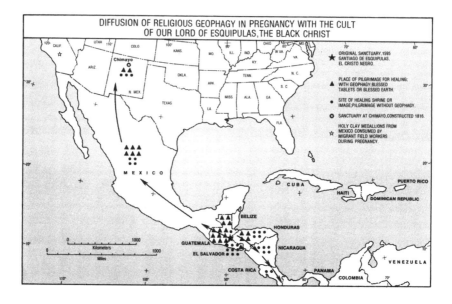

FIGURE 4.2
Diffusion of religious geophagy from Esquipulas, Guatemala (Hunter and Kleine 1984).
Reprinted by permission of *Geographical Reviews*.

trucks, private cars, and motorcycles awaiting the blessing of the vehicle and its contents.

Beyond Esquipulas: Chimayo

Religious geophagy in the Americas is not limited to Esquipulas. By the middle of the twentieth century, the Cult of the Black Christ had 55 places of worship and pilgrimage in seven countries; religious geophagy occurred at 26 of those places (De Borhegyi 1954; see also fig. 4.2). It would be tedious to describe each of the sites, but I cannot resist the description of at least one: Chimayo, New Mexico (fig. 4.3).

Chimayo is to holy earth what Lourdes is to holy water; it is the largest pilgrimage destination in the United States (Lamadrid 2001). Chimayo was considered sacred to Tiwa American Indians six hundred years before Christianity claimed it as its own in the 1800s, just as the site of Esquipulas was venerated before there was a church there. According to Tiwa cosmology, the sons of the Sun, the Twin War Gods, killed a giant that was

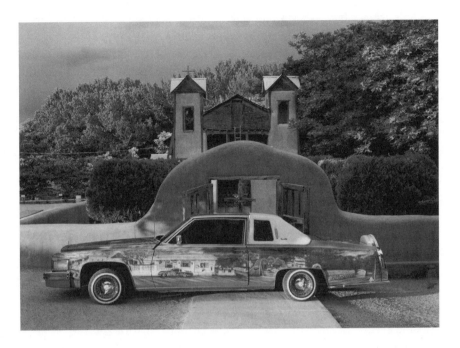

FIGURE 4.3
Lowrider Cadillac named "Chimayo," in front of El Santuario do Chimayo, New Mexico (1997). Photograph © by Craig Varjabedian. All Rights Reserved.

threatening the people. Fire burst from the earth at the site where he was killed, which caused the sacred spring to dry up, leaving only mud. The Tiwa used this mud to treat a number of health problems (Lamadrid 2001).

The source to which the sacredness of the earth at Chimayo is attributed has changed with the dominant religion, but the therapeutic function of the religious earth remains constant. To understand the Christian portion of the history of the healing earth at Chimayo, earth that is said to have helped to alleviate much physical and mental anguish, we must begin with someone who endured much self-inflicted pain: Don Bernardo Abeyta.[5]

In 1810, Penitente Bernardo Abeyta saw a bright light shining in the valley. He ran to the spot and dug to find the source of the light; a large crucifix appeared in the hole. He went to fetch the neighbors and the priest to show them the miracle. The priest carried the cross at the head of an ecstatic procession to the Spanish-built fortress church in Santa Cruz, five miles from Chimayo. He set the miraculous cross on the main altar and everyone went home for the night. The next morning, the cross was back in the hole from which Abeyta had dug it. After this happened several times, it became clear to even the priest (who wanted that miraculous cross in his own church) that the cross was meant to remain where it had first appeared. Penitente Abeyta began by building a small hermitage to house the miraculous wooden crucifix. He later received permission to build an actual chapel, Santuario de Chimayo, in 1816, where it still stands today (fig. 4.3).

The Sanctuary at Chimayo is the coziest religious site I have ever visited. A two-lane road winds through the New Mexico countryside and drops you, gently, in front of a broad adobe church nestled in a narrow mountain valley. The adobe makes it seem to radiate warmth even when it is blanketed in snow, as it was when I visited. The main part of the church, the nave, is decorated with carved wooden folk art, and the altar is crowned by a statue of our Lord of Esquipulas.

A small door on the left side of the church, near the altar, leads to a long, low rectangular room, filled with offerings and requests for miracles. Most compelling are the photos, of babies, children, adults, and the elderly, for whom a benediction or miracle has been asked. Letters and notes, some folded, some with their raw messages exposed, are tucked among the rosaries and framed images of saints. "Father, forgive me for my addictions." "If you cure my wife of cancer, I will never drink again." "Lord I will come here every year if you can please find a job for my daughter." "El Señor, please don't let my son die in Iraq."

One section of the low room is lined with proof that miracles do work: crutches and medicine spoons that are no longer needed, photos of loved ones who have been cured or returned from the streets, the war, or their addictions. Testimonials left at the shrine give thanks for divine help with surgery, illness, missing children, army service, marriage, conception, and eyesight. Signed prosthetic limbs are also hung in the room. In a tiny adjoining room at the furthest north corner is the source of the fervor: El Posito, the source of the holy earth. It's a small hole, roughly two feet in diameter, filled with fine sandy earth.[6]

Pilgrimages have been common since the construction of the church,[7] and many pilgrims still seek this earth for healing. About 300,000 pilgrims visit Chimayo every year, up to 40,000 during the last week of Lent alone. They come in many guises: gray-haired grandmothers, recent Mexican migrants, veterans of many wars, Protestants, testosterone-addled lowriders, devotional Aztec dancers, and New Age enthusiasts (Howarth and Lamadrid 1999; Lamadrid 2001). Some arrive at the church after walking for many miles; others roar up to the parking lot in their tricked-out rides. Between the reflector vests and rosary beads, do-rags and white Reeboks, leather jackets and oxygen tanks, it's a motley crew, but they seem cohesive, held together by their faith and purpose.

Jeff Sharlet, an American journalist, visited during the pilgrimage, and wrote:

> The day I visited, I witnessed people load the dirt into film canisters, plastic baggies, and paper envelopes. Some people simply wetted their fingers, dipped them in, and licked. One old woman turned to her husband for help getting the good stuff. "I can't bend down," she said, but he didn't seem to hear. "I can't bend down!" she shouted. Still no response. Finally, a younger woman scooped up a handful for the old lady, who reached down her shirt and rubbed it on her right breast—whether it was for cancer or an aching heart I was too shy to ask. She had a pinch left over, so she sprinkled it into her husband's hands. He rubbed it on his ears and smiled. (Sharlet 2002)

Islam

Christians are not the only ones who revere earth for its healing properties. The healing and protective power of earth procured from the tombs of Muslim saints is renowned. In early-twentieth-century Morocco, earth called *hanna* or *henné* was applied topically and made into amulets that could be worn, suspended in trees, and tucked into cupboards (Legey 1926). It reportedly cured the most intractable illnesses and protected the wearer from many other types of harms. Thieves, for example, would become blind, paralyzed, or even die if they stole objects protected by the holy earth.

The most famous earth associated with Muslim saints is that from the tomb of Imam Hussein, in Karbala, Iraq,[8] who was one of the adored grandsons of the Prophet Mohammed (Brugsch 1886). That particular earth is called *khak e shifa,* dust or earth of Karbala.

Dua are formulaic Muslim requests to God, and there are several that specifically involve the healing powers of this earth. When collecting *khak e shifa* the supplicant should recite the following: "Oh Allah I bind Thee by this clay and of that angel who had picked up this clay and of the Prophet through whom this clay was sent and of that vice regent who lies buried under this clay and ask Thee to shower Thy blessing on Mohammed (may peace be upon him) and Ahle Bait and make this clay a cure for all my diseases and a guardian against all fears."

When ingesting the earth, the *dua* to recite is: "In the name of Allah, for Allah, O Allah, the Lord of this sacred, helpful earth, the Lord of the light which is in it, the Lord of the body which is resting in it, the Lord of the guardian angels, let it cure my disease [*mention the name of the disease, then kiss the earth and eat it with some water and continue*], O Allah let this pure earth be a source of abundant means of livelihood, useful knowledge and a remedy for all my pains and ailments."

Hinduism

In some religions, earth is not sacrosanct, but important religious figures have ingested it. Take Krishna, for example. Purportedly born 3,000 years before Christ and frequently depicted as a little blue child, he has been worshipped by Hindus, Jains, Buddhists, and Bahá'ís. His attributes are many: a god-child, a prankster, a bride stealer, an uncle killer, a husband to 16,108 wives, a model lover, a product of immaculate conception, a divine hero, and . . . a geophagist. One day, one of the neighbors complained to Krishna's foster mother, Yashoda, that Krishna was eating dirt. Yashoda immediately went to him and told him to open his mouth; when he does, she gasps.

> She sees in Krishna's mouth the whole complete entire timeless universe, all the stars and planets of space and the distance between them, all the lands and seas of the earth and the life in them; she sees all the days of yesterday and all the days of tomorrow; she sees all ideas and all emotions, all pity and all hope, and the three strands of matter; not a pebble, candle, creature, village or galaxy is missing, including herself and every bit of dirt in its truthful place. "My Lord, you can close your mouth," she says reverently. (Martel 2001:55)

Hoodoo

Hoodoo, a predominantly African American cousin of voodoo, is a syncretic set of beliefs and practices, part folk religion, part magic, whose intent is to allow people access to supernatural forces to improve their daily lives. With so much rich symbolism to draw on, it is no surprise that hoodoo has some of the most enthralling uses of earth. Many uses are benevolent. For example, it can facilitate birth:

54

When a person is in labor with a baby an' dey don't have de baby, an' it seem dey can't have it, de ole lady dey had dey take de dirt dauber an' jest throw de nest—de whole business in right hot boilin' watah an' den took it off an' let it steep. An' den give it to de woman an' dat makes de lil' one come right out. Dat's whut ah heard about dirt dauber. (Hyatt 1970:432)

It can soothe a vexed mind:

I had a mother, she wus poison. Somebody took her hair. The fellah that come to cure her [. . .] told her to git up every night jist befo' midnight, she wus livin' in de country, an' walk to the fork of the road. She do that fo' five or six night. I don't know zackly how many nights that he told 'er but I know he told fer go to de fork of a road. He told fer take some dirt from under her front steps an' wear it aroun' her head as a poultice. He said that would help 'er. It helped a lot. (Hyatt 1970:437)

And just generally offer protection:

At de forks of the road—four forks of de road. Dey dig a hole and dey git red sand. Well, dat is fo' if anybody do anything to yo', yo' know, an' yo' boil it in water with lemons and yo' drink it. Dat is supposed to be if anybody do anything to yo' for bad luck. Jes' like yo' in bad luck—well, yo' do dat and dat is supposed to cut de bad luck off yo'. (Hyatt 1970:431)

So far, all the religious geophagy I have discussed has been used to achieve protection and health. In hoodoo, however, graveyard dirt is a common ingredient (fig. 4.4), and like fire or money, it can be used to achieve great good and great harm.[9] According to some, the most powerful stuff is that which is collected by the light of the smallest sliver of moon (Puckett 1926), but hoodoo practitioners have a multitude of approaches to collecting graveyard dirt (C. Yronwode, personal communication). According to the insert that came with graveyard dirt my mom bought for me at a candle shop in Detroit, graveyard dirt from a murderer's grave is carried to protect one against assassination, and graveyard dirt from an infant's grave is carried by pregnant women to insure an easy birth and heal the baby.

The punishment of adultery is one of the common nefarious uses for graveyard dirt.[10] In the blues song "Conjured," written by Esmond Edwards, a jealous woman sprinkles her lover's shoes with graveyard dirt and replaces his whiskey with embalming fluid in an effort to conjure him. However, retribution via graveyard dirt is not limited to (formerly) loved

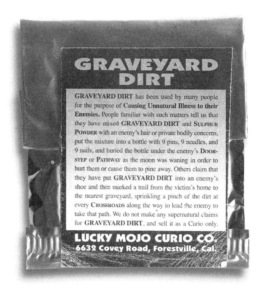

FIGURE 4.4
A package of graveyard dirt. Available for sale at www.luckymojo.com.

ones. For example, "If you get some dirt from the cemetery and put it in a box and place it under the steps of your enemy, it will cause trouble in their home" (Hyatt 1970:431). Extinguishing a black candle symbolizing the enemy by turning it upside down in a saucer of graveyard dirt can also spell their demise.

Noted author Zora Neale Hurston was an apprentice to Dr. Duke, a hoodoo practitioner in New Orleans whose specialty was law cases. She witnessed a number of uses of graveyard dirt to accomplish the feats his clients had asked of him (Hurston 1935: ch. 5):

> For that particular case [assault with attempt to murder] we went first to the cemetery. With his right hand he took dirt from the graves of nine children. I was not permitted to do any of this because I was only a beginner with him and had not the power to approach spirits directly. They might kill me for my audacity.
>
> The dirt was put in a new white bowl and carried back to the altar room and placed among the burning candles, facing the east. Then I was sent for sugar and sulphur. Three teaspoons each of sugar and sulphur were added to the graveyard dirt. Then he prayed over it, while I knelt opposite him. The spirits were asked to come with power more than

56

equal to a man. Afterwards, I was sent out to buy a cheap suit of men's underclothes. This we turned wrong side out and dressed with the prepared graveyard dust. I had been told to buy a new pair of tan socks also, and these were dressed in the same way.

On the day he came up for trial, Dr. Duke took the new underclothes to the jail and put them on his client just before he started to march to the courtroom. The left sock was put on wrongside out.

Hurston doesn't share the outcome of the trial with her readers, but with earth used for protection by so many, it once again illustrates the potency of belief.[11]

In this chapter, we have seen that people of many faiths acknowledge the powerful capacity of earth for religious reasons. From Israel to Guatemala, the United States to Iraq, consecrated earth is believed to bring about desired changes, be it conception, recovery from a chronic illness, or faithfulness in a lover. These happy results are a stark contrast to the subject of the next chapter—unhealthful outcomes of non-food consumption.

CHAPTER FIVE

Poisons and Pathogens

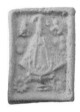 AS WE saw in the last chapter, earth clearly has a place in the treatment of both physical and metaphysical problems. But earth and other pica substances have also been suggested to be the cause of a number of sicknesses, including **anemia,** poisoning, and parasites. In this chapter, we return to what is clearly demarcated pica behavior, the purposive ingestion of craved non-food substances, and explore its purported negative consequences from a much more biomedical point of view.

Anemia

Pica is associated with anemia far more frequently than it is with any other negative health condition. I would estimate that there are twenty case reports of anemia associated with pica for every one report of any other negative health outcome.

Anemia, simply put, is a condition in which **hemoglobin** concentration is too low. Hemoglobin is a protein with many vital functions, and one of its most important is transporting oxygen to cells throughout the body. Thus, a deficiency of hemoglobin means that red blood cells are not getting enough oxygen. Because oxygen is necessary for aerobic metabolism, people with anemia become easily tired. This presents a major problem in places where daily activities involve much physical exertion, like fetching water, chopping firewood, and pounding grain. There are other, more dire consequences of anemia than fatigue. One of these includes poor blood coagulation, which is especially dangerous for pregnant women because it can cause them to bleed to death during delivery. There are many less overt consequences of anemia that are still very serious, including increased risk of infection and poor cognitive function. These consequences adversely affect quality of life, shorten the lifespan, and hinder economic output.

The World Health Organization estimates that more than two billion people are anemic. Because anemia is so widespread and because it has so many negative health consequences, it is considered to be a major public health issue (Stoltzfus 2001). Yet most people who are anemic don't know it; it is not readily detectable until it becomes severe. The classic symptom of anemia is pallor, and that usually doesn't occur until anemia is moderate or severe.[1] Iron molecules in the heme portion of the hemoglobin molecule make your blood look red. If hemoglobin concentration is insufficient, blood is thinner and less red. An anemic person can therefore appear pale, particularly where skin is thinnest, e.g., the membranes of the eyes, the palms of hands. In extremely severe anemia, blood can even appear watery.

Many conditions can cause anemia. It can be caused by blood loss, e.g., heavy menstrual periods, hookworm infection. Red blood cell destruction, such as that which occurs during an episode of malaria or during chemotherapy, can also cause it. So can insufficient red blood cell production, which can be due to inadequate intake or absorption of micronutrients or genetic disorders called **hemoglobinopathies**, e.g., thalassemia and sickle-cell disease. Iron deficiency causes at least half of the anemia worldwide, but other micronutrient deficiencies can too, including folate, vitamins A and B12, and zinc.

There has also has been much discussion about pica as the cause of anemia; the two are frequently associated (cf. Appendix E). This association was first written about in 30 A.D. by a Roman physician, Cornelius Celsus: "They who, without jaundice, have a pale complexion for some considerable time, are plagued with pains of the head or have a morbid appetite for earth" (Celsus/Grieve 1756). It has since been remarked upon throughout medical history. Physicians treating plantation slaves did perhaps the most to popularize the belief that pica "breaks the texture of the blood entirely" (Browne 1756:64). By the nineteenth century pallor was often considered to be a symptom of pica.

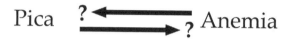

FIGURE 5.1
The causal arrow in the relationship between pica and anemia has been pointed both ways. While some have stated that pica may cause anemia, others suggest that anemia may cause pica.

The diagnosis [of pica] May be nearly formed from the pallid appearance of the lips, the gums and the whole membranous lining of the mouth, and from the condition of the tongue, which in health performs its duty with so much alacrity, lying bleached and bloodless, scarcely able to represent the motives of its owner. (Cragin 1835:357)

The association between anemia and pica was noted throughout the world, however, and in Tanzania the overlap was so large that Dr. David Livingstone ("I presume") mistranslated *safura*, the Swahili word for *anemia*, as "the disease of earth-eating" (Livingstone and Waller 1875:346). In a journal entry dated November 29, 1870, while visiting Zanzibar, he wrote:

Safura is the name of the disease of clay or earth eating, at Zanzibar; it often affects slaves, and the clay is said to have a pleasant odour to the eaters, but it is not confined to slaves, nor do slaves eat in order to kill themselves; it is a diseased appetite, and rich men who have plenty to eat are often subject to it. The feet swell, flesh is lost, and the face looks haggard; the patient can scarcely walk for shortness of breath and weakness, and he continues eating till he dies. Here many slaves are now diseased with safura; the clay built in walls is preferred, and Manyuema women when pregnant often eat it.

Typically, a causal relationship between pica and anemia has been declared even in the absence of sufficient scientific data (e.g., Crosby 1976a,b). Pica is usually blamed for anemia, i.e., people become anemic after eating these items. The causal arrow has also been pointed in the opposite direction (fig. 5.1). Some people think that being anemic or "not having enough blood" causes people to eat items that are typically not considered to be food. In fact, one of the first times a Pemban explained to me why they ate earth, she told me, "We eat this stuff because it gives us what we need to build our blood." The relationship between pica and anemia is a rich one; it will be discussed at length in chapter 8.

Heavy Metal Poisoning

Pica can be a source of lead poisoning. Lead, the softest, heaviest metal, is highly toxic. With each exposure to lead, more of it accumulates in our body, in our hair, and in our teeth, causing a variety of neurological, gastrointestinal, and reproductive problems. Acute lead poisoning causes seizures, comas, and death. Lead poisoning is particularly scary because most of it happens without warning (except for the kind of lead poisoning inflicted by Wild West gunslingers). Lead poisoning is also linked to anemia, since lead interferes with hemoglobin synthesis.

Lead has found its way into many craved non-food substances—earth, paper, chalk, glazed pottery, and powder—because it is incredibly useful from an industrial point of view. Leaded paint and leaded gasoline have been particularly insidious vectors of lead poisoning.[2] Leaded gasoline meant that lead was found anywhere that cars emitted exhaust, especially in roadside earth. Indoors, painted walls eventually flake, and those lead-laced flakes work their way into household dust. Outdoors, flakes of leaded paint work their way into backyard soil.

It was a major public health victory in the United States when lead was banned from paint in the 1970s (Lourie 1971) and gasoline in the 1980s. With so much less ambient lead, there was a concurrent decrease in the prevalence of elevated blood levels in the United States (from 77.8% to 4.4% between the 1970s and 1980s [1997]). However, there are thousands of new cases of elevated lead levels in the United States alone every year (Meyer et al. 2003), most of which are attributed to pica behavior. This association is not unique to us. A search in the PubMed database will turn up hundreds of articles from Australia, India, Great Britain, Japan, and France reporting a strong relationship between pica and lead poisoning. The incidence of pica among lead-poisoned populations has been reported to be as high as 62% (Berg and Zappella 1964), 83% (Conrad 1979), and 94% (Tanis 1955). Most of these cases are children and pregnant women. For example, in a 2002 study of lead poisoning among pregnant New Yorkers, 39% of women with elevated blood lead had engaged in pica (Klitzman et al. 2002). In several instances, the source of lead poisoning of a neonate confounded clinicians until they realized that it was the mother's taste for ground pottery (with leaded glaze) that had transmitted the lead to the infant (Hamilton et al. 2001; Lowry et al. 2004; Mycyk and Leikin 2004).

Lead is not the only toxic substance that those who engage in pica can ingest. Soil can be contaminated with all sorts of harmful compounds, such as mercury drudged up from gold mining in the area (Campbell et al. 2003) and radioactivity from a Superfund site (Harper et al. 2002; Simon 1998). Other soils have been shown to contain persistent organic pollutants including banned neurotoxins (Dean et al. 2004) and cyanide and phenol (Calabrese et al. 1999).

When soils are tested for safety, exposure levels are calculated based on accidental ingestion (licking your fingers, dust on your apple), not on purposive consumption of several grams (Calabrese et al. 1999). Therefore, recent soil tests might not be indicative that "your" geophagic earth is safe. For example, a 2004 study of clays sold to be mixed with water and used for naturopathic healing in Italy indicated the presence of varying levels of heavy metals; the authors of the study urged regulation of such products that included establishment of potential toxicity for the consumption of quantities larger than accidental consumption (Mascolo et al. 2004).

Seemingly innocent pica substances can also be toxic. One woman slowly poisoned herself with mercury by consuming the pages of a novel (mercury is a fungicide in paper pulp) (Olynyk and Sharpe 1982). Other pica substances may just contain too much of a good thing. For example, humans need small doses of copper, potassium, and fluoride, but some soils have very high concentrations of these and cause hypercupremia (too much copper) (Holt et al. 1980), hyperkalemia (too much potassium) (Abu-Hamdan et al. 1985; Garg et al. 2004; Gelfand et al. 1975; Hussey 1975), and fluorosis (too much fluoride) (Fisher et al. 1981), respectively.

And then there are a few people who crave more overtly toxic substances. Examples here include mothballs (which contain naphthalene or 1,4-dichlorobenzene) (Anziulewicz et al. 1959; Fisher et al. 1981) and matchheads (which are extremely high in potassium) (Abu-Hamdan et al. 1985; Armstrong and Kourany 1979; Smulian et al. 1995).[3] Such cravings in the general population are far, far more rare than those for earth, starch, and ice.

Geohelminths

Parasites, roughly speaking, are pretty much anything that take more than they give. Leeches, fleas, and tapeworms are all well-known examples. Geohelminths (*helmis-*, Greek for "worm") are another common group of parasites that belong to the phylum Nematoda and include roundworms, hookworms, and whipworms. They live in the dirt (thus the geo-) and do not need an intermediate host to infect you. There are two main pathways by which people become infected with geohelminths. One is the oral-fecal route (swallowing eggs that have been shed in an infected person's feces, typically through contaminated food or water). The other route is transdermal (they crawl through your skin). Because residence in the earth is part of their life cycle, it's easy to see why geohelminths have long been associated with geophagy.

Geohelminth infection is not pretty. The life cycle of *Ascaris lumbricoides*, the large intestinal roundworm, is particularly gruesome. Once you swallow roundworms, they crawl through your intestines into your bloodstream and circulate until they reach your lungs. This is where they mature. Once they are big enough, they cause their host to cough them up, at which point he or she swallows some of them, and they grow larger in the intestine and begin to shed eggs. The eggs that pass out of the body will wait in the earth for the next unwitting host to ingest them, and the whole process begins anew.

Although it is never fun to be parasitized, sharing hard-won nutrients with hundreds of 25 cm long roundworms— especially if you are a child or a pregnant woman who really needs them—is particularly serious because it can have devastating effects on health and growth. On top of outright thieving your nutrients, they can irritate your gut, which inhibits absorption of nutrients. They can also cause bleeding at the site of attachment, which causes a further drain of nutrients. Hookworm, in fact, is one of the biggest infectious causes of anemia today (Stoltzfus et al. 1997). Other roundworms repay their host by wiggling through the organs ("visceral migrans"), sometimes popping through your eyeballs and inflaming your brain. All this is to say that parasites are not a good thing.

And yet these parasites surround us. Viable geohelminth eggs are waiting in much of the dirt around the world, especially in places where open defecation by their hosts occurs.[4] Thus, it is understandable that, for a long time, it was thought that pica, especially geophagy, increased the likelihood of geohelminth infection (e.g., Anell and Lagercrantz 1958; Hooper and Mann 1906). It was an appealing idea, for it would also help to explain the frequent association between pica and anemia: people eat earth, become infected with hookworms, and become anemic.

However, we now know that the ingestion of non-food substances cannot explain the bulk of hookworm infection, the most common geohelminth in humans (Geissler et al. 1998a; Gelfand 1945; Saathoff et al. 2002; Vermeer and Frate 1979; Young et al. 2007). Why not? Hookworm is most infectious transdermally, not through ingestion. They burrow under your finger- and toenails and are merrily on their way to your intestines. The soils geophagists select also make it less likely that they transmit hookworms. Larvae do not survive well in the clayey soils preferred by most geophagists, and if they do, they are generally killed by the sunbaking, air drying, and heating that many geophagists do to their soil prior to consumption (cf. chapter 1).

The jury is still out on the contribution that geophagy makes to roundworm and whipworm infections. Several types of roundworm infections have also been attributed to the consumption of earth upon which furry four-legged friends have trodden, including dogs, cats, and raccoons (Glickman et al. 1981; Good et al. 2004). Studies among schoolchildren in Jamaica (Wong et al. 1991), South Africa (Saathoff et al. 2002), and Kenya (Geissler et al. 1998a) indicate a higher prevalence of roundworm and whipworm among those children who ate earth; no differences were found in a similar study in the United States (Vermeer and Frate 1979). In Pemba, we found no differences between roundworm and whipworm infections by geophagy behavior (Young et al. 2007; this study is described in more detail in chapter 6). Furthermore, we were unable to detect any eggs of these parasites in the pica samples we analyzed. The differences observed between our study and the others is likely attributable to the fact that our study was done among pregnant women; the others were done among children. Adults were more likely careful with the collection and preparation of soils than were the children.

In short, at this point it's clear that pica does not contribute to the geohelminth infection with the largest public health consequence: hookworm. Pica's role in the transmission of other geohelminths has not been studied well enough to draw any sweeping conclusions.

Other Physical Damage

In addition to being a vector for the aforementioned poisons and pathogens, pica substances have been known to seriously damage most parts of your alimentary canal, from teeth to anus.

Dental Damage

Dentists can identify some geophagists the same way they identify bulimics: by the wear on their teeth. Front teeth chip while nibbling hunks of clay, and molars wear down by grinding bagfuls of ice. One woman wore out several pairs of dentures with her ice-crunching (Coltman 1971). Several members of the Yahoo! Cornstarch Discussion Group crunch on pumice stones from Target, which cannot be easy on the pearly whites. Notably, they all came up with the idea to eat pumice independently.

Parotid Gland Swelling

The parotid gland is a chicken nugget–sized gland in your cheek that secretes saliva, the first step in the digestion of starches. If you have a lot of starch to digest, say if you are eating two boxes of Argo starch a day, your parotid gland has a lot of secreting to do to get that starch digested. Thus, it is no surprise that several cases of swollen parotid glands have been reported among starch consumers (Greenberg 1977; Merkatz 1961; Silverman and Perkins 1966).

Gastrointestinal Issues

The bulk of the reported physical damage done by pica has occurred in the gastrointestinal tract. Gastroliths are, literally, rocks in your stomach. They are normal in animals that use stones to help grind their food, such as herbivorous birds, crocodiles, and alligators. They are not normal in humans, but through their consumption of excessive amounts of pica substances (e.g., multiple boxes of cornstarch per day), people have created gastroliths in their gut that need to be surgically removed (e.g., Allan and Woodruff 1963).

Occasionally, severe constipation can result from earth-eating (e.g., Courbon et al. 1987; Robinson et al. 1990). A handful of fecal impaction cases, where the bolus of feces is stuck and just will not move forward, have been reported (Holt and Hendricks 1969; Wrenn 1989). Fewer still are the cases of intestinal obstruction (Anderson et al. 1991; Key et al. 1982), where *nothing* can move in the gut. Rarer still, and more dangerous, is perforation of the intestines (Amerson and Jones 1967; Graham 1976).

The frequency of intestinal issues that result from pica is difficult to determine because (a) people may show up for care without admitting that they have been engaging in pica, (b) they may self-treat the milder intestinal disturbances, and (c) we do not know what the denominator is (i.e., how many people are engaging in pica) to be able to calculate a percentage of how many wreak havoc on their alimentary canal.

On the bright side, one physician has suggested that there could be an advantage to slower intestinal motility: it allows more time for nutrients to be absorbed (Oke 1972). This seems unlikely, since most pica substances are typically consumed in small quantities (cf. chapter 1) that are not sufficient to slow the passage of food through the gastrointestinal tract. Furthermore, pica substances are not usually eaten before a meal, but afterwards, or as a snack throughout the day, so they would not be holding up any material to be digested and absorbed.

Sexual Maturity

Geophagy has been associated with delayed sexual maturation in Turkey and Egypt (Prasad et al. 1961; Say et al. 1969). A number of children and adolescents there have been diagnosed with a syndrome of iron deficiency anemia, dwarfism, hypogonadism (underdeveloped sexual organs), and zinc deficiency; most of them also ate earth.

Obesity

Although most pica substances contain no calories, cornstarch does. A one-pound box of cornstarch contains 1,680 "empty" calories (i.e., pure energy) with little protein, vitamins, or minerals. (As a reference, it takes about 3,500 calories to gain one pound.) Although we don't know how frequently this occurs, some people do eat boxes of this stuff every day (cf. chapter 1), which can easily add up to many pounds. Obesity presents many health problems under normal circumstances. It causes unnecessary stress on your bones, joints, heart, and circulatory system, and increases your risk of diabetes, cancer, stroke, heart disease, and death. And during pregnancy, when most pica occurs, excess gestational weight gain also increases the risk of negative outcomes for the fetus.

In short, pica is strongly associated with anemia, and sometimes associated with heavy metal poisoning and non-hookworm geohelminth infections. It can also wreak havoc on the alimentary canal. For these reasons, pica has been considered a pathological behavior by most medical professionals (Reid 1992). In contrast, we have also seen that pica substances are associated with medicines, health, and healing (chapters 3 and 4). Thus, it is clear that pica is associated with both positive and negative conditions. But *why* pica? Turn now, dear reader, to part II, which deals with this very question.

66

But Why?

CHAPTER SIX

Dismissal and Damnation

*A Historical Perspective on the
Purported Causes of Pica*

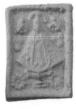 WE SPEND a lot of effort avoiding dirt. We scrub under our nails, launder our clothes, rinse our vegetables, and sweep the floor. It is therefore understandably jarring to hear that some people seek out a substance whose presence others try to eliminate.[1] If cleanliness is next to godliness, where does that put geophagists in the divine order?

Indeed, the stigma of eating earth is reinforced by the Old Testament. After all, geophagy was among the first (Judeo-Christian) divine punishments. When Adam and Eve were kicked out of the Garden, Adam was punished with hard work, Eve with labor pains, and the snake with crawling on his stomach and eating dirt. Unkind references to eating dust are made throughout the Bible, usually with references of abject humiliation.[2]

Disdain for dirt is reinforced by the English language, where it is regularly demonized. "Dirt" is the damning details you have on someone that can ruin their reputation, or marriage, or both. According to the online Urban Dictionary, *dirt* is also criminal activity, low-quality marijuana, and "a person that is low on the social ladder, either because of unfettered promiscuity, poor personal hygiene, or any other indicator of social status" (Urban Dictionary 2009). A "dirt nap" has not ended well for the napper. "Dirt-eater" is used to taunt the Tauron race in the 2010 science fiction television series *Caprica*. And dirty jokes are something to hide from children, nuns, and parents.

Despite these negative connotations of dirt in Western culture, the absolute *outrage* expressed about pica is frequently incommensurate. When I describe the phenomenon of pica to those who have not heard of it, some reactions are frequently orders of magnitude more emphatic than I could have ever expected, spanning shock, horror, and disgust. Similarly, in quite a bit of ethnographic literature, descriptions of pica (mostly geophagy) are adjacent to passages about deviant behavior including cannibalism and aberrant sexual behaviors. One particularly graphic article about sexual practices in Zanzibar describes the variety of "perversities" in which the local population engages: straight prostitutes, gay prostitutes, transvestites, sex toys, bestiality, sadism, masochism, and . . . geophagy (Haberlandt 1899).

The problem is that "dirt" and "earth" or "clay" have been conflated conceptually. This conflation is responsible for much of the very visceral response. Sometimes it's revulsion, nails-on-the-chalkboard style. Other times its fascination, gawking-at-a-tragedy style. Either way, the fear-and-loathing responses over the last centuries have left little mental space to wonder if there could be any advantage to this behavior; too much time has been spent damning or dismissing those who engage in it. But what if pica is somehow beneficial, and not due to a flaw in morality, culture, or physiology?

The purpose of this chapter is to describe how, for centuries, pica has been considered to be a behavior that is at best useless, and at worst injurious. You will read about the six groups of people who have historically been described as engaging in pica. The flawed rationale behind the condemnation is discussed for each group. Information about the frequency, duration, and severity with which pica has been condemned makes it possible to surmise why pica has been so readily dismissed until the twentieth century. I wrap up by recounting more recent judgmental reactions to pica, which leads to a discussion of other reasons why pica may be concealed as well as suggestions for establishing a more accurate estimate of pica behavior.

Once we understand why and how pica has been dismissed, we are in a better position to consider alternative explanations, ones that consider potential adaptive functions. Therefore, this chapter also provides a launching point for the rest of the book. By exposing flawed explanations of pica, it becomes easier to identify where we should focus our scientific efforts, i.e., the most promising explanations worthy of our best scientific efforts, the hypotheses outlined in chapters 7, 8, and 9.

Let us turn now to the six groups who have historically been associated with pica: indigenous populations, slaves, pregnant women, poor whites in the southeastern United States,[3] children, and the mentally ill.

"The natives"

There are literally hundreds of accounts of pica among indigenous populations throughout the Americas, Africa, Asia, and Oceania. Primarily, they have been written by anthropologists, missionaries, and explorers who came to study, convert, or exploit them, and they represent some of the most judgmental descriptions of geophagy. (Harsh judgment was, of course, not reserved uniquely for pica; these populations were condemned for most aspects of their daily life.)

Most authors seemed unable to fathom any rational reason for the consumption of earth. For example, of his exploits around the Zambezi in Central Africa, Sir Harry Johnston, a British colonial administrator, wrote that "in some districts there is a craving for argillaceous clay, which they eat with (I imagine) results that are eventually fatal" (Johnston 1897:436). It is of note that in the preface of the book, Johnston includes a picture of a white linen–clad table in the middle of a jungle, flanked by two servant boys, and captioned "My table in the wilderness." It seems safe to conclude that he had, at best, a cursory acquaintance with local daily life.

Yet despite their social and cultural distance from local people, many explorers felt comfortable attributing non-food consumption to cultural inferiority. In the Peruvian Amazon, geophagy was taken as evidence that "the natives appear to be sunk in an abyss of moral filth and depravity from which nothing but a strong tide of European immigration can lift them" (1873). In Vietnam, pica was considered "a deprivation of taste, maintained by local tradition" (Hamy 1899). In the West Indies, it was described as "the filthy habit of eating dirt" (Duprey 1900). There are many more such examples.

Slaves

Non-food cravings have been reported among slaves in Africa as well as enslaved populations of African origin in Brazil, the Caribbean, and the United States. Pica was not confined to one age group or gender: "dirt-eating respects neither age nor sex" (Cragin 1835). They predominantly ate

71

earth, but when that was not available they would consume plaster, ash, limestone, cloth, and paper (Mason 1833).

The greatest outrage against pica is found in this literature. The indignation on the part of slave owners and the physicians who treated them likely stemmed from the belief that pica damaged their financial interests.[4] "Nothing is more horribly disgusting, nothing more to be dreaded," wrote one plantation owner in Jamaica (Roughley 1823:118–19). *Cachexia Africana*, the term most frequently used for pica at that time, was "more destructive and lamentable than any other to which negroes are liable" (Williamson 1817:266). The death and destruction that slave owners attributed to pica is well illustrated in a 1909 letter that Lieutenant Colonel J. A. Wyllie wrote to *Scientific American*, opposing the need for laws for humane treatment of slaves. After describing how "the Angolan in the native state is an absolute animal—he has neither home nor family—please grasp this fact firmly," he explains how the real cause of the health problems seen among slaves is *not* the lack of humane treatment of slaves by their owners but alcoholism and geophagy, which "account for more than 90 percent of the black mortality in the Island [of São Tomé, to which many Angolans were shipped]" (Wyllie 1909).

Because the perceived "invariable fatality" (Imray 1843) of cachexia Africana reportedly caused the abandonment of plantations (e.g., Carpenter 1844; Imray 1843), slave owners were anxious to understand and stem the death toll due to this disease. As such, the causes of pica among slaves in the Americas were reported extensively in nineteenth-century medical journals; slave owners were desperate to know how to limit what they understood to be a very damaging behavior to their property. Many explanations were given for pica:

Physicians in the British West Indies claimed pica was caused by *licentious behavior*. "Those dissolute and irregular in their habits—such as indulging to excess in dancing during the night, promiscuous intercourse with those of the other sex, &c. The passion of jealousy should also be mentioned as predisposing to the disease in both sexes" (Imray 1843:306).

Breastfeeding and prolonged *lactation* were also thought to be culprits. "The child becomes accustomed to too much tenderness, unsuitable to its station, giving it a fretful longing for the mother, and her scanty milk, engendering disease, and what is worse than all, often giving it a growing liking for the hateful, fatal habit of eating dirt" (Roughley 1823:118). Similarly, another physician wrote that the "erroneous method of nursing negro children is by far the most frequent cause of dirt-eating" (Maxwell

1835:413). Of course, it is now well established that breastfeeding is one of the best gifts a mother can give her baby.

An alternative explanation was *imitation*:

Negro children are noted for the aptitude with which they imitate the manners and actions of their associates [such that there are] frequent opportunities of observing how rapidly the propensity for eating dirt spreads through a vigorous healthy gang of children from the example and persuasion of an incorrigible juvenile offender." (Maxwell 1835:414)

This, of course, does not explain the origins of the behavior.

These descriptions of lustfulness and breastmilk prompting geophagy are far-fetched enough to scoff at. However, the most common explanation of geophagy among slaves is a sobering one: suicide. Many physicians thought that pica reflected "discontent with their present situation and a desire of death in order to return to their own country" (Hunter 1788:311). "Large groups of Negroes indulged in excessive dirt-eating due to a firm belief that after death, they would return to their native homes" (Maxwell 1835:428).

Although *suicide* was indeed a way to end their existence as slaves, it is unlikely that geophagy was a method for ending their lives. There are many accounts of slaves desperate enough to hang themselves, drown themselves, and even swallow their tongue to hasten their end (1846; Courlander 1976). Further evidence that controverts the suicide hypothesis is that in at least some settings, slaves went to a good deal of trouble to prepare the clay for eating by baking it (Mason 1833).

Nevertheless, convinced that geophagy was destroying their property, slave owners meted out unspeakable brutality when slaves were caught eating pica substances. One torturous method for controlling pica was the use of a metal mask (figs. 6.1 and 6.2).[5]

As curative means, neither promises nor threats (even when put in execution,) nor yet the confinement of the legs and hands in stocks and manacles, exert the least influence; and their preventative effect is as temporary as their employment; so great is the depravity of the appetite, and so strongly are the unfortunate sufferers under this complaint subjected to its irresistible dominion. A metallic mask or mouthpiece, secured by a lock, is the principal means of security for providing against their indulging in dirt-eating, if left for a moment to themselves, nor does this effect a cure or save the life of the patient. (Cragin 1835:299–300)

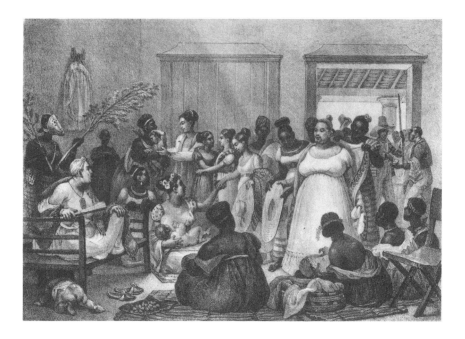

FIGURE 6.1
Depiction of a Brazilian slave being punished for her alleged attempt to end her life through geophagy (at far left of image). The original caption reads: "Behind the mistress of the house is one of the young female slaves, charged with the boring work of hunting flies and cousins, by waving tree branches. She offers an example here to the European of proof of unhappiness of her captivity with the spectacle of the tin mask wrapped around the face of this victim, a sinister indication of the resolve she had to kill herself by eating dirt" (Debret 1835:47).

The use of masks on slaves to prevent pica has even found its way into modern fiction: an insipid, pandering romance novel, of all genres. In *A Respectable Trade*, a slave who has given herself the name Died of Shame becomes pregnant after being raped by Sir Charles, a white slave trader. When Sir Charles is told of her geophagic behavior by her owners, Frances and Miss Cole, he is quick to prescribe "a bridle" for her (Gregory 2007:154–56).

"She will not eat food . . . She is eating . . ."
"Earth?" he guessed.
Frances's glance flew to his face. "You knew?"
He shrugged. "It's not unusual. A foul habit, isn't it? The women do it often. It makes them sick as dogs. They get the yaws, and they will eat it

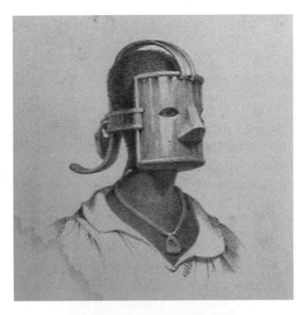

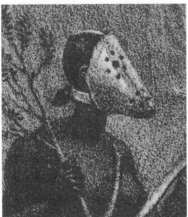

FIGURE 6.2

Drawing of a slave wearing an inhibitive metal mask. The caption on this plate reads: "Negro Heads, with punishments for Intoxication and dirt-eating. . . . The mask is a punishment and preventative of . . . dirt eating" (Bridgens 1836). *Bottom photo*: slightly enlarged version of iron mask depicted in figure 6.1.

till they die sometimes. It is their mad spite. They know they are robbing you of their purchase price. They are insane with spite. You will need to use a bridle, ma'am."

"A bridle?"

He tutted in irritation. "Of course, you will not have one to hand. I had thought myself at home! We put a bridle on them when they eat soil. A metal cage which goes around the face, under the jaw, with a gag of metal across the mouth. Their driver must take it off at mealtimes and watch her to make sure she eats her food. She must wear it all the rest of the time. They are cunning as monkeys. If they want to eat dirt, they will get their hands on it somehow. The only way is to gag their mouths."

In Jamaica, when masks failed to thwart pica, corpses were even decapitated:

What could not be effected by any of the means just mentioned has been in part accomplished upon some estates, as I have been informed, by cutting off the heads from the dead bodies of those who have died of this vicious practice. The negroes have the utmost horror and dread of their bodies being treated in this manner, and the efficacy of this expedient, which can only operate upon the mind, is a strong proof that the disease in its origin is more a mental than corporeal affection. (Hunter 1788:313–14)

"The weaker sex"

As we saw in chapter 1, pregnant women are the group most likely to indulge in pica (cf. Appendix B). Pregnant women are, of course, famous for their cravings. As a little girl, I was convinced that pregnancy would be nothing but bliss because it was a period when I could *finally* order my loved ones to fetch the foods of my heart's desire, whatever they may be.[6]

In many cultures, it is considered important to indulge a pregnant woman's cravings, no matter how unreasonable. In the nineteenth century, in parts of Germany and Italy, for example, "pregnant women might, if they liked and without being liable to punishment, satisfy their desires for game, fruit and vegetables even if they belonged to other people" (Ploss et al. 1938:456–57). In Toni Morrison's *Song of Solomon*, Pilate, a woman very knowledgeable about the matters of birth, concurs: " 'When you expectin, you have to eat what the baby craves,' Pilate said, 'less it come in the world

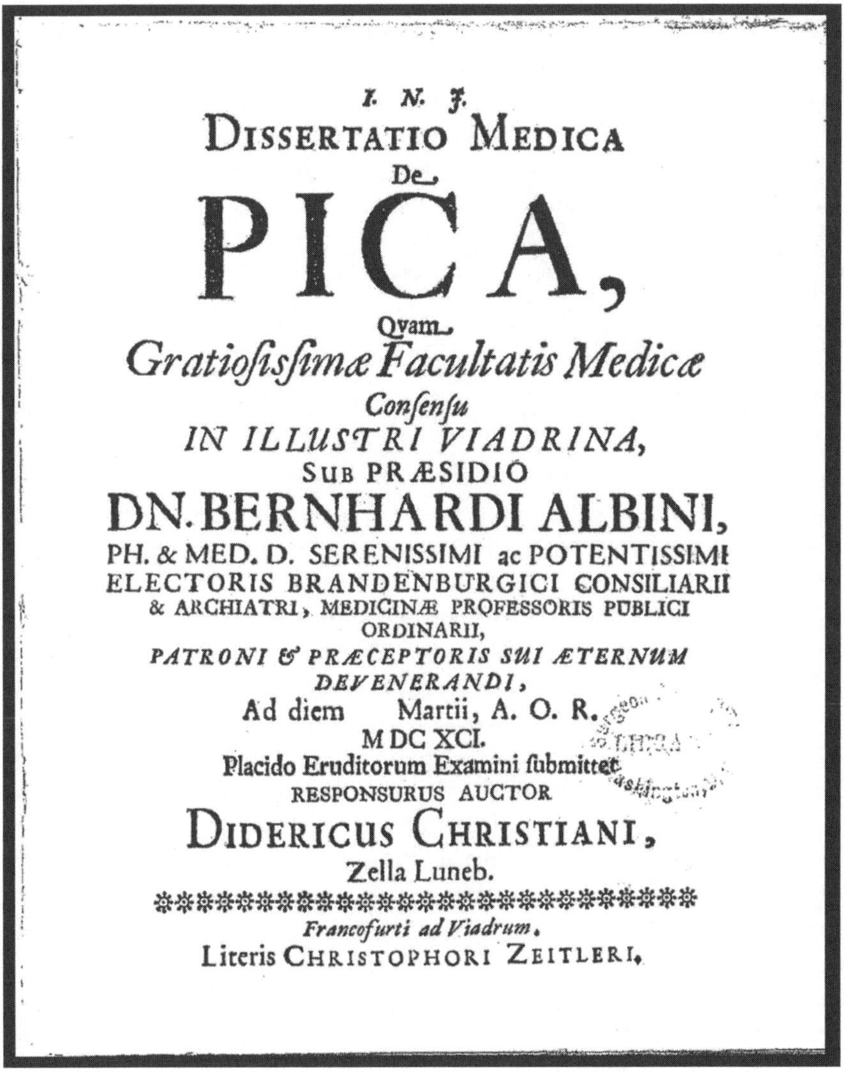

I. N. J.
DISSERTATIO MEDICA
De
PICA,
Qvam
Gratiosissimæ Facultatis Medicæ
Consensu
IN ILLUSTRI VIADRINA,
SUB PRÆSIDIO
DN. BERNHARDI ALBINI,
PH. & MED. D. SERENISSIMI ac POTENTISSIMI
ELECTORIS BRANDENBURGICI CONSILIARII
& ARCHIATRI, MEDICINÆ PROFESSORIS PUBLICI
ORDINARII,
PATRONI & PRÆCEPTORIS SUI ÆTERNUM
DEVENERANDI,
Ad diem Martii, A. O. R.
M DC XCI.
Placido Eruditorum Examini submittet
RESPONSURUS AUCTOR
DIDERICUS CHRISTIANI,
Zella Luneb.
Francofurti ad Viadrum.
Literis CHRISTOPHORI ZEITLERI.

FIGURE 6.3
One of approximately 25 *dissertatios* written about pica by physicians in the 17th and 18th centuries (Christiani 1691).

hongry for what you denied it' " (Morrison 1987:131–32; see also Appendices B and D).

The indulgence of pregnancy cravings is even what got Rapunzel locked in her tower. According to the tale, a pregnant woman noticed some greens planted in her neighbor's garden and longed for them to the point of death. As her dutiful husband was returning home with the greens for her, the enchantress neighbor caught him. He begged for mercy, and the old woman agreed to let him free, if their unborn child was given to her at birth. Desperate, the man agreed. The enchantress named her Rapunzel and whisked her away to a tower with only one room and one window, where, as you know, she was stuck until she let down those lovely locks.

In short, pregnant women are permitted culinary transgressions that others are not. Explanations for their causes have varied over the centuries. Just as colonialists attributed pica among indigenous societies to cultural inferiority, Renaissance doctors attributed longings for non-food items to the mental and physical inferiority of women (fig. 6.3). In literature from this period, pica was very much considered a "woman's disease" and was described in book sections with this very heading. Sometimes, the general nature of our souls was to blame. Pica was attributed to our "impotence of spirit" (Christiani 1691) or the fact that "the soul in this sex is not seen (at least in many) to reach a sufficient degree of perfection so that it may resist luxuries" (Betten 1687). "We warn the female sex, as being weaker, of this evil [pica] which is familiar and peculiar to them" (Maler 1692:6). At other points, pica was attributed to the physical inferiority of our female constitution, pregnant or otherwise, e.g., "menstrual spirit titillates nerves of the belly which in turn affects the brain" (Maler 1692) and "a great collection of crudities in the stomachs and parts adjacent, and these humors when they grow worse cause the Pica" (Riverius et al. 1663).

In later years, the "deranged" cravings commonly understood to be a part of pregnancy made it easy to dismiss any possibilities of non-food cravings as somehow making sense. Instead, they were just part and parcel of us lunatic pregnant women.

Sandlappers

Geophagy among European settlers in the southern United States dates to 1709 (Lawson 1967 [1709]) and was widespread enough to become the basis of slurs for poor white residents from West Virginia to Florida: "hillbillies," "sand-hillers," "sandlappers," and "clay-eaters" (Bradley 1964;

78

Buck 1925; Welch 2008).[7] By all accounts, these unlanded, uneducated whites eked out a miserable existence that included tattered clothes, drafty shacks, moonshine, and geophagy. Although there are fewer reports of pica among this population than among slaves, this is probably due to the fact that "masters procured for their slaves far more medical inspection than poor whites procured for themselves [although] the vicious practice was as common among the whites" (Phillips 1929:347).

A fictionalized account of life in the South during the Civil War era based on a New England author's travels there vividly captures the abysmal living conditions of poor whites and the race and power dynamics between the three social classes. In this passage, a black servant and his English master discuss the living conditions of a poor rural Georgian family with whom they spent the night due to inclement weather (Gilmore 1862:82–83).

As we rode along I said to the driver, "Scip, what did you think of our lodgings?"

"Mighty pore, massa. Niggas lib better'n dat."

"Yes," I replied, "but these folks despise you blacks; they seem to be both poor and proud."

"Yas, massa, dey'm pore 'cause dey wont work, and dey'm proud 'cause dey'r white. Dey wont work 'cause dey see de darky slaves doin' it, and tink it am beneaf white folks to do as de darkies do. Dis habin' slaves keeps dis hull country pore."

"Who told you that?" I asked, astonished at hearing a remark showing so much reflection from a negro.

"Nobody, massa; I see it myseff."

"Are there many of these poor whites around Georgetown?"

"Not many 'round Georgetown, sar, but great many in de up-country har, and dey'm all 'like—pore and no account; none ob 'em kin read, and dey all eat clay."

"Eat clay!" I said; "what do you mean by that?"

"Didn't you see, massa, how yaller all dem wimmin war? Dat's 'cause dey eat clay. De little children begin 'fore dey kin walk, and dey eat it till dey die; dey chaw it like 'backer. It makes all dar stumacs big, like as you seed 'em, and spiles dar 'gestion. It 'm mighty onhealfy."

"Can it be possible that human beings do such things! The brutes wouldn't do that."

"No, massa, but dey do it; dey'm pore trash. Dat's what de big folks call 'em, and it am true; dey'm long way lower down dan de darkies."

There are plenty of firsthand accounts of geophagy among poor southern whites to substantiate this fictionalized one. They ate clay "with gusto, as if it was a piece of meat or boiled potato" (1866). Mrs. Jefferson Davis, wife of the president of the Confederate States of America, described clay eaters as "wretchedly poor, ignorant, and with . . . complexions the color of the clay which they ate to satisfy their starved bodies" (Sinclair 1957:7). Others described how the cabin served as both shelter and food since the mud mortar was frequently nibbled upon, and how there were entire areas designated for the excavation of geophagic earth (Cotting 1836).

Dirt-eating "became the mark of poor white depravity most dwelt upon by Northern and foreign observers" (McIlwaine 1939:57). They were lambasted for it just as slaves and indigenous people were: "with the tenacity of ignorance these people cling to their filthy habits, traditions and superstitions" (1897). In 1866 a correspondent for the *New York Times* even described them as "the lowest representatives of the United States I have seen—little more than mere animals. [. . .] Their habits of the most filthy and repulsive character. [. . .] Strange undeveloped, repulsive creatures they. Do they and the Platos and the Dantes and the Shelleys of the race represent the same species?"

The stereotype of Southerners as geophagists continues today. Roy Blount Jr., a fabulously witty author who grew up in Georgia, was asked about the verity of a 1986 *New York Times* article (Eckholm 1986) about geophagy at an urbane soirée (Blount 1988:48).

The very night of the dirt-eating story, I was in someone's chic salon eating arugula. A woman with a crew cut heard my accent.

"What do you do?" she asked.

I said I was a writer.

"Ah, yes," she said. "Of course. Southerners are all natural storytellers. Sitting on the old screen porch, dog under the rocker, flies on the baby, everyone spitting and spinning yarns compounded of biblical cadences and allusions to animals named B'rer.

"One thing I never realized, though," she went on, "was that you eat dirt."

At that point there were two tacks I could take. I could say, "Well, I know there are some folks down South who like to chew on clay, but I never ate any myself and neither did any of my relatives or friends, and in point of fact, I never even saw anybody eat dirt."

The response to that tack would have been a knowing look. "Here is a man who comes from people who eat dirt, and he thinks he is better than they are." She would be thinking I couldn't handle stigma. Or that I was inauthentic. Southern and inauthentic: the worst of both worlds.

So I took the second tack. "Hell, yes, we eat dirt," I said. "And if you never ate any blackened red dirt, you don't know what's good. I understand you people up here eat raw fish."

He then decided to raise money to open a geophagic restaurant and collected $3,800 for that purpose in just one evening.

Children

There is plenty of evidence of children's penchant for pica. Some of it is purely anecdotal. In recalling the great culinary moments of his life, the American author Guy Davenport reminisces about a visit to the home of his black nurse, who had muttered, "what this child needs is a bait of clay."

The eating took place in a bedroom, for the galvanized bucket of clay was kept under the bed, for the cool. It was blue clay from a creek, the consistency of slightly gritty ice cream. It lay smooth and delicious looking in its pail of clear water. You scooped it out and ate it from your hand. The taste was wholesome, mineral, and emphatic. I have since eaten many things in respectable restaurants with far more trepidation. (Davenport 1980:137)[8]

Other anecdotal evidence of American kids loving dirt is that Binney & Smith had to change the name and smell of their Magic Scent Crayola brown crayon. They had already altered the recipes and smells once because too many children were eating the crayons; Licorice had become Leather Jacket, Apricot became Lumber, and Chocolate became Dirt. Only Dirt was apparently attractive enough to ingest, such that Binney & Smith had to revamp yet again.

In addition to these anecdotal stories, there have also been several scientific studies of the prevalence of pica in children in America (see Appendix C). These were prompted by the high prevalence of lead poisoning purportedly due to the consumption of lead-infused soil, paint, and paper. Many of them were conducted in inner-city areas, and as such, pica was taken as an indication of the depravity of inner-city life (Cohen et al. 1965), and again dismissed.

There have been far fewer studies of the prevalence of pica among children than among adults, and these have occurred in a much more narrow geographic setting. The few studies of prevalence that have been conducted among children do, however, make it clear that children outside the United States engage in pica, especially in Africa. The prevalence of geophagy, typically in the form of earth from termite mounds, was higher in each of the four African settings than it was in all but one study in the United States. If queries were made about the prevalence of pica in other countries, I'm sure that more would be revealed.

Is short, the relative frequency of this behavior among children has not been regarded as a clue to potential functionality; instead, it has been the grounds for discounting it. After all, as they say, they are *just children.*

The Mentally Disturbed

The final aberrant explanation of pica is that it is a result of a range of mental anguish, from minor calamities to serious psychoses. One of the most memorable dramatis personae in the cast of fictional pica characters is Rebeca from García Márquez's *One Hundred Years of Solitude* (cf. Appendix D). She arrives at the house of the Buendía family as a traumatized 11-year-old orphan, with her parents' bones clattering in a bag.

> They could not get her to eat for several days. No one understood why she had not died of hunger until the Indians, who were aware of everything, for they went ceaselessly about the house on their stealthy feet, discovered that Rebeca only liked to eat the damp earth of the courtyard and the cake of whitewash that she picked off the walls with her nails. (46)

Later, as a teenager, she falls madly in love with the pianola instructor, Pietro Crespi. When he leaves Macondo, she is utterly lovesick:

> She would put handfuls of earth in her pockets, and ate them in small bits without being seen, with a confused feeling of pleasure and rage, as she instructed her girl friends in the most difficult needlepoint and spoke about other men, who did not deserve the sacrifice of having one eat the whitewash on the walls because of them. The handfuls of earth made the only man who deserved that show of degradation less remote and more certain, as if the ground that he walked on with his fine patent leather

boots in another part of the world were transmitting to her the weight and the temperature of his blood in a mineral savor that left a harsh after-taste in her mouth and a sediment of peace in her heart. (69)

In the world outside of novels, it has been suggested that pica functions as a soothing behavior, associated with childhood memories of one's own mother engaging in pica (Corbett et al. 2003). Of course, this does not explain why the behavior disappears in adolescence and why mothers (and not fathers) ever engaged in pica in the first place, and then, primarily during pregnancy.

Pica is occasionally a feature of a range of much more severe mental problems, including obsessive-compulsive disorder, autism, schizophrenia, and developmental impairment (Beecroft et al. 1998; Danford et al. 1982; McAlpine and Singh 1986; McLoughlin 1988; Roosendaal and Weits-Binnerts 1997). There have even been cases of non-food items removed from the stomachs of people with schizophrenia dramatic enough to make international headlines, such as an elderly woman who had swallowed £175.32 ($650) in loose change (Beecroft et al. 1998).

Although such pica is clearly a distinct phenomenon from your comparatively run-of-the-mill taste for clay or cornstarch, the consumption of non-food items by the mentally disturbed has caused people to lump the behavior of all consumers with that of the mentally unwell.

Concealment of Pica Today

Clearly, centuries of condemnation and punishment have been heaped on those who crave and eat non-food substances. This stigmatization has real consequences for our understanding of pica: those with a taste for clay (or baby powder or newspaper or plaster) go to great lengths to *avoid disdain* by hiding it: this has occurred the world over, from India to the Caribbean, and everywhere in between. "I have surprised them while they still had remainders [of earth] in their mouth, between their teeth, or on their tongue, and despite this evidence, they exclaimed loudly that I was wrong, that they had never even had the idea . . . of eating earth" (Levacher 1840:255).

Although in the 21st century the grounds for any proclamation of pica as "good" or "bad" remain limited, harsh judgment continues (Henry and Kwong 2003). For example, in a 2005 interview with the *New York Times*, the director of the Scientific Center of Hematology in Kyrgyzstan was quick to revile it: "You'll go straight to the devil if you eat this clay" (Wilensky-Lanford 2005). Even modern academic literature contains descriptors like "bizarre," "perverted," "morbid," "disgusting," and "unnatural."

Posts in 2009 on the Yahoo! Cornstarch Discussion Group corroborate the concealment of pica:

> I have been addicted for 7 years and I have no one to talk to about this. I hide it from my boyfriend because he thinks its just something I should be able to stop doing in the blink of an eye.

> i have hidden it from my family for 15 years. i dont know wut i would do if they found out. i guess i would have to stop then. i would be so ashamed. if it werent for living with my family, i think i would be consuming cornstarch baby powder 24/7.

I MAKE DAILY STOPS TO WALMART FOR CHALK AND HIDE THE BOXES WHEN I GET HOME

Pica receives similar disdain in popular media. Take, for example, *The Tyra Banks Show*. Tyra introduced the episode (entitled "Bizarre Eating Habits") by turning to her audience and warning: "They eat things that will totally shock you!" As her guests recount their cravings—baby powder, chalk, cornstarch, and clay—she exclaims "What!?!?!" as the camera pans to audience members clucking and shaking their heads.

Besides fear of judgment, there are other reasons why people hide pica. One of these is the implications of dirt-eating. In areas where pica is understood to be a sign of pregnancy (cf. pp. 15–16), admitting to geophagy is tantamount to being pregnant, and in some places, including Pemba, pregnancy is something to be kept secret. Therefore, *modesty* can motivate the denial of pica.

Another reason why people conceal pica is out of *reluctance to appear poor*. I returned to Pemba two years after we completed the large epidemiological study of anemia and pica (described in chapter 2) to do some follow-up work. Shufaa, a Pemban woman who came to our house to prepare delicious Swahili food, had been a participant in that study. She also regularly provided commentary on our research activities. One day, she came out of the kitchen just as a research assistant and I were discussing why Mama Hamisa, who had admitted to eating earth two years ago, was now denying that she had ever even tasted it. Shufaa explained:

Even I didn't tell the researchers that I was eating earth when you asked me about it for your study. But I did! Yep, my husband bought me some when I was first pregnant and he told me to eat it, so I ate it. I didn't tell you that because I didn't want you to think we didn't have anything else to eat.

Back to Mama Hamisa. I ran into her at the market several weeks later. She told me that she had in fact engaged in pica, but that she remembered that she had only after her mother had reminded her. She apologized profusely for forgetting. So, it seems, pica behavior is easily *forgotten* once cravings have ceased.

Sometimes, pica is underreported not because it is concealed or forgotten, but because those who are documenting nutritional or medicinal or pregnancy-related behaviors simply *do not know to ask*. In the preface, you read how I stumbled upon pica by accident. This is the case for many researchers. One of my favorite examples of accidental discovery of pica involves a physician who saw a patient and her family celebrating a birthday in the clinic. Much to the physician's surprise, red Georgia clay was served, baked and topped with butter and salt (Kraemer 2002). Among the Tiv of Nigeria, a geographer wrote how "even medical missionaries who have worked among the Tiv for years have been unaware of the custom despite its apparent universal practice within the tribe" (Vermeer 1966:197). There are many more such examples (e.g., Cooksey 1995; Grigsby et al. 1999; Hooper and Mann 1906; Rainville 1998).

The risk of overlooking pica is compounded by the fact that pica does not easily fit into a *conceptual category*. People may think of pica substances as medicine, a food additive, or "just a craving," such that dietary recall questions about what a person has consumed in the last week or month do not probe with appropriate prompts.

This great variation in societal attitudes is sure to affect the likelihood of a person engaging in pica, as well as the likelihood of their admitting they do so. One way to think of the interaction of the cultural environments on behavior is through the concept of **effect modification**. An effect modifier is not a cause of outcome Y per se; rather, it modifies the effect of X on Y (fig. 6.4). If phenomenon X is a cause of pica, cultural attitudes are an effect modifier that may decrease or increase the likelihood of pica actually being manifested. For example, I may feel like eating chalk, but when I turn on the television and see the ridicule heaped on Tyra's guests, I'm likely to feel inhibited. Conversely, effect modifiers can magnify pica, too. It might not

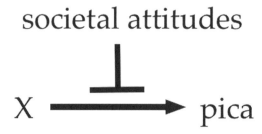

FIGURE 6.4
An example of effect modification: societal attitudes can both magnify or inhibit the manifestation of pica.

have otherwise occurred to me or to Shufaa to eat clay during pregnancy, but because her mother, aunts, and neighbors did, and her husband bought her the clay, the idea became more palatable.

Establishing Accurate Estimates of Pica Behavior

There are thus many reasons for an observer to miss pica. How, then, to establish accurate estimates of its prevalence? In research settings, I use several strategies to reduce underreporting. First, I begin interviews about pica by describing how non-food cravings are a mystery to scientists, and how no one really knows if they are unhealthy or not. This means that *the interviewee* is the expert on pica, and the truthfulness of their answers will make an important contribution to science. If research assistants have engaged in pica, they will describe their own pica habits at the beginning of the interview. This helps to normalize the behavior. It's also best to ask about pica in a private setting, i.e., one in which a woman feels comfortable discussing intimate subjects, including her pregnancy status. Pica behavior should be asked about prospectively, i.e., at the time it could be occurring, rather than retrospectively, i.e., asking about pica behavior last month, last year, five years ago, etc. Finally, to reduce the chance of false negatives, I phrase questions about the consumption of pica items as *how much* of the substance they eat, rather than *if* they eat it.

Furthermore, it is necessary to get the right people to ask the questions—people of the same sex and of similar ethnic background, preferably without much social distance. For Beverly Dunston's dissertation research about pica among black women in New York City, four graduate students in nursing pilot-tested her forms in the same population (Dunston 1961). The three black female interviewers heard a lot about pica, but the white male interviewed no one whom admitted to pica. Another example of probable underreporting comes from Mississippi. Interviews done by a black midwife revealed a prevalence of pica of 57% among non-pregnant women, while only 28% of pregnant women (whom we know are more likely to engage in geophagy) "admitted" to it during interviews with male interviewers of unspecified race, one of whom was from outside the community (Vermeer and Frate 1975; Vermeer and Frate 1979).

Throughout this chapter we've seen how pica has been dismissed as aberrant—natives lost without the saving grace of European culture, slaves seeking an escape from their miserable lives, pregnant women suffering from humors, children who know not what they do. The purported inferior culture, physiology, intellect, and/or morality of each of these groups has made it easy for privileged white male explorers, scholars, and physicians to dismiss pica, or worse, qualify it as an aberrant behavior that demonstrates the righteousness of the white patriarchal social order. Perhaps if upper-class white men had engaged in pica more frequently it would be less demonized. But they don't (or at least haven't admitted to it), so we are left with some lively, befuddling, and horrifying descriptions of this practice among "others." This attribution of pica to the consumers' physical, mental, or spiritual inferiority is one of the primary reasons why pica received little scientific attention until the twentieth century.

Concealment is the other main reason for the dismissal of pica. Concealment of pica continues today, to avoid disdain, to preserve modesty, to avoid appearing poor, because consumers forget, because scientists don't know how to ask, or because they don't ask in a way that consumers can understand.

Fortunately, this is changing, as you will see in the next few chapters.

CHAPTER SEVEN

Pica in Response to
Food Shortage

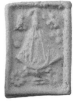OUR DIET is intimately associated with the earth. Accord-
ing to an ancient Chinese proverb, we owe our very existence
"to a six-inch layer of topsoil and the fact that it rains."
Or, as Tom Robbins puts it, "Dirt is the mother o' lunch"
(1984:260). Implicit is that the earth *yields* food, not that
the earth *is* food. But some have suggested that there is a less
circuitous path between the land and our sustenance: direct consumption.

In many creation stories, earth was all there was to eat at the beginning
of the world. A touching Polynesian legend from the Cook Islands tells of
a husband and a wife who lived "very very long ago" (Ellis 1853:65–66).
They had only one son whom they loved dearly, but he was delicate and
sickly. At that time, the only food was *araea*, a red earth, but their son was
too weak to eat it. The husband was so distraught to see his child wasting
away that he decided to die to become food for him. He prayed to the family gods, and in the evening he called to his wife and said, "I am about to
die. Take my body and plant it. When you hear a sound like that of a leaf,
then a flower, then an unripe fruit and then of a ripe round fruit falling on
the ground, know that it is I, who have become food for our son." She soon
heard these sounds, and the next morning she took her son out to see a
large beautiful tree with shining leaves and loaded with breadfruit (fig. 7.1).

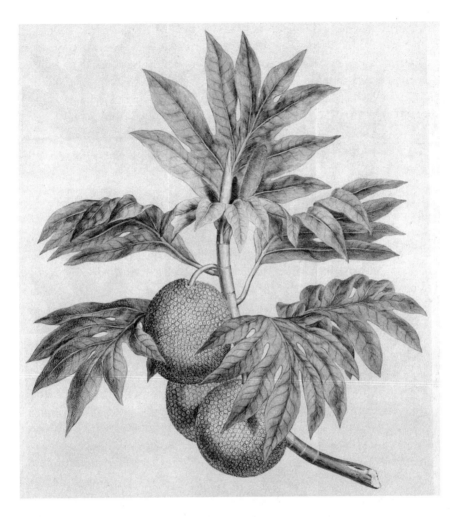

FIGURE 7.1
A branch of the breadfruit tree with the fruit. Drawing from John Hawkesworth, *An Account of the Voyages Undertaken . . .* (1773).

They brought the first fruit to the family god, the second to the king, and then roasted and ate the breadfruit for themselves and never ate clay again.

In this chapter, I will present examples of earth used during famines. I will then explore and evaluate the first of the two nutritional explanations of pica—that pica is a response to hunger—using data from many sources, including the Pica Literature Database and our study on Pemba.

Earth as a Famine Food

Earth has been eaten the world over when other foods were not available. Fictional evidence of this is found in Pearl S. Buck's *The Good Earth* (1994[1931]). Earth is highly symbolic throughout the novel: the acquisition of land permits Wang Lung (the protagonist Chinese peasant farmer) and his family to ascend from abject poverty to live like royalty; the earth is the medium through which he pays tribute to his ancestors; and, as he and his family near starvation, earth quells the hunger pains of his children.

> The extreme gnawing which he [Wang Lung] had had in his stomach at first was past and he could stir up a little of the earth from a certain spot in one of his fields and give it to the children without desiring any of it for himself. This earth they had been eating in water for some days—goddess of mercy earth, it was called, because it had some slight nutritious quality in it, although in the end it could not sustain life. But made into a gruel it allayed the children's hunger for some time and put something into their distended, empty bellies. (84)

Geophagy has been documented during a number of actual famines in China (Biot 1839; Mallory 1926; Martini and Grothe 1910; Torrette 1836; Yang et al. 1904). One French missionary in China described a famine followed by a flood, followed by a plague, that caused many once rich men to sell their houses, their farming equipment, and finally their wives, daughters, and sons. In this terrible period, white clay procured from a mountain was highly valued as food (Torrette 1836:85).

China is not the only place where earth has been eaten as a substitute for food. During the Thirty Years' War (1618–1648), Germany faced such terrible food shortages that people began to mix white earth with flour, and baked bread out of this mixture (Strose and Suhle 1891:7). There were unforeseen fatal consequences of this geophagy: the hill where people collected this clay collapsed and killed five villagers. **Diatomaceous earth**, or kieselguhr, was eaten during various sieges of the fortress of Wittenberg, Germany, in the eighteenth century (Buschan 1930). During a famine in Lapland (Scandinavia), diatomaceous earth called *bergmehl* (mountain meal) was mixed with flour and tree bark and baked into bread (Dahms 1897; Hopffe 1917; Schmidt 1871). Earth was also eaten in periods of hunger in Siberia, Finland, and Italy (Hopffe 1917). According to at least one scholar, in the United States some people have been hungry enough to eat dirt for it to become part of the American slang, i.e., "dirt-poor" (Den Hollander 1935).

Hunger has been a favored explanation of geophagy by colonial explorers in Oceania, the Americas, and Africa. For example, La Billardière, a French explorer in New Guinea, wrote, "I should never have imagined that cannibals would have recourse to such an expedient when pressed by hunger" (1800:214). The famed German explorer Alexander von Humboldt attributed some of the earth consumption by Amazonian Indians to hunger (1821), as did Arctic explorers, e.g., "the natives eat this earth in times of scarcity" (Richardson 1851).

Hunger continues to motivate some geophagy in the 21st century. In 2008, for example, there were all kinds of food crises due to sharply increasing food prices (a result of rising fuel costs, food crops diverted to biofuels, and hurricane damage). One of the many consequences of these crises, at least according to several reporters, is that the only consumables some Haitians could afford were *bonbons terres*, or earth cakes (Bourne 2008; Katz 2008).

> The mud has long been prized by pregnant women and children here [Haiti] as an antacid and source of calcium. But in places such as Cité Soleil, the oceanside slum where Charlene shares a two-room house with her baby, five siblings, and two unemployed parents, cookies made of dirt, salt, and vegetable shortening have become a regular meal. "When my mother does not cook anything, I have to eat them three times a day," Charlene said (Katz 2008).

Similarly, in Sierra Leone, women in 2008 were regularly eating smooth white clay balls that were once solely consumed during pregnancy (Brunhuber 2008). Aisha Jalloh is one such woman. She explained how normally they were only consumed to make the baby strong and remove "bad water" from the stomach during pregnancy. "When I ate it [while pregnant], the vomiting stopped." But it has become a regular food for her. "Sometimes when I'm hungry, I will eat this because of poverty," she said. "It helps sustain my life."

Testing the Hunger Hypothesis

There is clear evidence that some people are eating things they do not consider to be food when they are hungry. But how much pica is motivated by hunger? The next section examines the four predictions that stem from the hypothesis that hunger is a response to food shortage (see Appendix G):

Prediction 1. People eating non-food substances have little other food to eat.

Prediction 2. People would feel less hungry after eating pica substances.

Prediction 3. Pica substances would not be desired when "typical" food was available.

Prediction 4. Almost any non-food item would be eaten by the consumer.

Prediction 1: People Eating Non-food Substances Have Little Other Food to Eat

If hunger motivated pica, we would expect people who engage in pica to have little else to eat. The easiest way to test that prediction is, of course, to simply ask if they are hungry. When this is not possible, either because observations of pica were made without measuring food availability or because questions about food availability are likely to elicit untruthful answers, food availability can be indirectly measured. This can be done by measuring the consumer's wealth (e.g., income, assets, food stores), determining if there are food shortages caused by natural disasters or normal seasonal fluctuations, and assessing if they have experienced recent weight loss.

In the Pica Literature Database, we located data on hunger status in 72 cultural reports in which earth was consumed (fig. 7.2). Among these, geophagy was attributed solely to hunger in only 16 reports (22%). This proportion may even overestimate the importance of hunger, because some authors seemed unable to fathom any reason for the consumption of earth other than hunger.

In 20 reports (28%), earth was sometimes eaten out of hunger. In these instances, it was described as being eaten for "pleasure," "custom," "craving," or "habit," as well as due to food shortages, in the same populations. Such was the case with von Humboldt's description of Otomac people living along the banks of the Amazon: "If the Indians eat earth from want during two months (and from three quarters to five quarters of a pound in

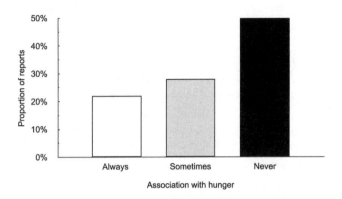

FIGURE 7.2
Frequency with which hunger was associated with geophagy in 72 cultural-level reports in the Pica Literature Database.

twenty-four hours), he does not the less regale himself with it during the rest of the year" (1821, pt. 2, pp. 639–64). In other words, clay is eaten almost exclusively during the two months that typical food is not available, but it also continues to be eaten throughout the year. Similarly, as described above, in Haiti and Sierra Leone people have turned to earth as food, but its provenance and alternative function is to quell the malaise of pregnant women. Even when observers declared that hunger was the cause of geophagy, they provided evidence that contradicted their conclusion. For example, upon landing in New Caledonia, La Billardière describes how one of the locals "came up who already had his stomach well filled, but who nevertheless ate in our presence a lump of very soft steatite of a greenish color and as big as his two fists" (1800:214). The satiety of this man did not prevent La Billardière from concluding, on the very next page, that geophagy was motivated by hunger.

Some observers were explicit that earth was never eaten for lack of food (the third column in fig. 7.2). For example, while describing pica in slaves in the southern United States, Buckingham wrote, "they do not take the clay here as substitute for food, since they are never without an abundant supply" (1842:551). During his travels in West Africa, David Rutherford showed children of the Camaroon ethnic group some geophagic clay used by the Batanga people (Rutherford and Distant 1881:468). They "eagerly besought me to give them some," and when he did, "they greedily swallowed it, afterwards expressing a desire" for more. He goes on: "These children had just supped, and their evident appreciation of the clay could, therefore, hardly be connected with hunger, and would seem to indicate an appetite, or at least a liking, however unnatural, not much related to the desire for food."

When the hunger levels of the populations observed were not explicit, the adequacy of the food supply of geophagists was indirectly indicated. For example, David Livingstone wrote how "rich men who have plenty to eat are often subject to it" (Livingstone and Waller 1875:346). Elsewhere, the obesity of Mississippi geophagists (Vermeer and Frate 1979) and the elegantly dressed Spanish nobility who consumed clay pots called *bucaros* (Gautier and McQuoid 1853:89) all point to unproblematic procurement of calories.

In our study on Pemba we asked pregnant and non-pregnant women and men directly about the circumstances that prompted amylophagy and geophagy, including if hunger was an impetus. It never was (Young et al. 2010a). In case people were concealing their hunger (which happens more often than you might think), we also asked about indicators of economic status, the number of meals, and the variety of food they ate. There were no differences in these economic indicators by reported pica behavior.

A final piece of evidence that contradicts this prediction is that some pica substances are actual food ingredients that have not yet been cooked. The consumption of uncooked rice in Pemba is a good example. Only a very small proportion of potential energy is available from raw rice and some of the other typical amylophagy items, such as flours and raw potatoes (cf. chapter 1, n. 6, p. 172). If food is available, eating it in a form in which few calories are available is not consistent with this prediction.

Prediction 2. People Would Feel Less Hungry After Eating Pica Substances

A second prediction of the hunger hypothesis is that enough non-food items would be eaten to assuage the consumers' hunger. This is difficult to gauge; in ethnographic reports, specific quantities were rarely mentioned. Sometimes, phrases were used such as "a few morsels" (Maupetit 1911), "size of a nut" (Garnier 1871), "egg-sized lump" (Whiting 1947), and "chewed in small quantities" (Morel-Fatio and Tobler 1896), all of which indicate small amounts. In 11 of the 361 reports of geophagy in the Pica Literature Database, the amount of earth consumed was actually weighed; 30 grams was the modal reported intake. If you cup your hand, 30 g of dry earth or uncooked rice is about enough to fill your palm up to where your fingers begin.

These quantities are consistent with more precise reports in recent biomedical studies of geophagy in Africa, which have recorded daily consumption of 20–40 g of earth per individual (Geissler et al. 1997; Luoba et al. 2005; Saathoff et al. 2002). On Pemba, the mean amount of raw rice consumed was 34.5 grams per day and for earth, 26.5 grams per day (Young et al. 2010a).

Now, can 30 grams fill the belly? Look at your cupped palm again. It does not seem like a palmful could sate an individual. But remember, these are dry items that can absorb a lot of water. Smectite, for example, is a type of clay that can expand up to 30 times in volume. Rice, too, swells in liquid. It is thus possible that eating small quantities of highly absorbent items can give a feeling of satiety that hungry people so desperately want, even if it provides little nutrition.

Prediction 3. Pica Substances Would Not Be Desired When "Typical" Food Was Available

If hunger motivated pica, we would not expect the substances to be strongly desired, but rather eaten as a desperate remedy for hunger. Accordingly, we would not expect phrases like "a devouring passion" (Galt 1872) and "great attachment" (Shannon 1794) to be used in conjunction with pica. But they were two hundred years ago, and similar terms are still used today (see also chapter 1, "A devouring passion"). For example, in 2002, Alabaman Carrie Webb said, "I used to tear up a bank. When I used it regular, I don't care what it done. I went wild over it, I ate so much. I was killin' that dirt" (Spencer 2002). The Pica Literature Database contains other data indicative of the desire for pica. Among the 77 cultural reports that included descriptions of consumers' feelings toward geophagy, 93% mentioned a very strong desire or craving for it.

In short, the fondness that pica consumers have for their substance of choice is remarkably strong, and not at all consistent with a last-resort dish, as this prediction implies. Many people love this stuff.

Prediction 4. Almost Any Non-food Item Would Be Eaten by the Consumer

If people are simply looking to stop the rumbling in their stomach, many nontoxic substances and certainly most earths would do. Yet we did not find a single report of indiscriminant geophagy in the Pica Literature Database; people always chose their earth very carefully. Similarly, in Pemba, people were very selective about their pica materials (Young et al. 2010b). This should be no surprise; you've already read about the great lengths people go to for their pica: the long car drives, the expensive icemakers, the secrecy with which "their" source of earth is protected. Therefore, it seems that people seek something from their non-food consumption beyond filling a void in their stomach.

In conclusion, there is little to substantiate this hypothesis. Although consumers may feel more full after engaging in pica (consistent with Prediction 2), they frequently have other food to eat (contradictory to Prediction 1); pica cravings occur when typical food is available (contradictory to Prediction 3); and pica substances are extremely carefully selected (contradictory to Prediction 4). While hunger has motivated a small fraction of non-food consumption around the world, it is safe to say that it does not explain the bulk of pica.

So what does?

CHAPTER EIGHT

Pica as a
Micronutrient Supplement

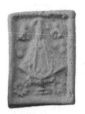 IN *THE GRAPES OF WRATH*, Rose of Sharon, preg-
nant and husbandless, is pessimistic about the outcome of
her pregnancy; she and her family are enduring the dust
bowl and the Great Depression, among other hardships
(Steinbeck 1967:368). As she complains to her mother about
how she wishes there was milk for her to drink, she pops
something in her mouth.

"I see you nibblin' on somepin. What you eatin'?"

"Nothin'."

"Come on, what you nibblin' on?"

"Jus' a piece a slack lime. Foun' a big hunk."

"Why, tha's jus' like eatin' dirt."

"I kinda feel like I wan' it."

Ma was silent. She spread her knees and tightened her skirt. "I know,"
she said at last. "I et coal oncet when I was in a fambly way. Et a big piece
a coal. Granma says I shouldn'."

Slack lime is a form of calcium oxide used in whitewash, plaster, and
mortar. The timing of Rose of Sharon's consumption of calcium-rich non-

food as she longs for calcium-rich food nicely embodies the second of the two nutrition-related hypotheses about pica—that pica serves as a dietary supplement. A similar explanation of pica also emerges in this focus group discussion among several Sioux Native Americans (Reading 1982).

> I craved dirt and I had all kinds of vitamins that my doctor gave me.
> I used to like that white dirt.
> Like you put in log houses?
> Yeah!
> You eat that stuff because you have a lack of something.
> Minerals.
> Yeah, a lack of minerals.

The idea here is that the mouthfuls of earth or chalk or starch contain the micronutrients in which the consumer is deficient. The supplement hypothesis is an appealing one because it is both intuitive and straightforward. For this hypothesis, the micronutrient that has had the most attention paid to it is iron—because of the association between pica and anemia—but zinc and calcium have also been suggested as substances the consumer is seeking to augment in the diet. Supplementation is by far the most popular explanation of pica, and many scientists have been absolutely convinced of its truth (e.g., Crosby 1976a,b; de Castro and Boyd-Orr 1952; Külz 1919). "In actuality it is the consequence [of anemia], and the patients reach for such earth from an inner necessity, instinctively, as one says. They reach for that earth that is useful for their blood deficiency" (Külz 1919:42). Other scientists remain skeptical. One even warned that "anyone venturing dogmatic assertions on this subject may end up eating his words (logophagia), or—if he is a betting man—his hat" (1969).

This chapter explores the possibility that a micronutrient deficiency motivates pica. There are three predictions that can be made from this hypothesis (see Appendix G); each will be examined in turn:

Prediction 5. Pica would be associated with a micronutrient deficiency.
Prediction 6. Pica would be associated with populations with the highest micronutrient requirements.
Prediction 7. Elimination of the deficiency would cause pica to cease.
Prediction 8. Pica substances would provide micronutrients in which the consumer is deficient.

For each prediction, I will group supporting data as they relate to iron, zinc, and calcium deficiencies.[1] One warning: the data for testing this hypothesis are not ideal. Sample sizes are small, methodologies are not consistent, and some analytical techniques are now outdated. Bearing these limitations in mind, however, you will see that there is still a lot we can learn from the last few centuries of observations and the last few decades of experiments.

Testing the Micronutrient Supplement Hypothesis

Prediction 5. Pica Would Be Associated with a Micronutrient Deficiency

You read in chapter 5 that the association between anemia and pica is at least two thousand years old (p. 59). It is also very well documented. I have filing drawers crammed with hundreds of case studies of pica and micronutrient deficiencies. For the most part, these reports are a blur of dense, clinical data in which the non-food items consumed, micronutrient deficiency symptoms exhibited, clinical tests performed, and results of interventions drone on and on and on. But some stick out, such as the anemic woman whose geophagy was "discovered" because of the soil sediment in her colostomy bag (Stevens 1993). And the case report from the seventeenth century in which a physician treated an extremely pale 13-year-old girl who had pica with the thermal waters at Bath, England (Peirce 1697).[2] And the dissections of the still-warm bodies of slaves with "watery blood," in which the state of the internals from the brain to the colon are described in great detail (Telford 1822). And the severely anemic child who ate the paper label from the iron drops she had been prescribed, but consumed very little of the actual iron supplement (Buchanan 1999). The common thread among these many case reports from all over the world is that micronutrient deficiencies feature prominently. This is, of course, consistent with Prediction V.

Now, the problem with these case studies is that while they tell us that pica exists among people who have been cared for and written up by medical professionals, we cannot know the prevalence of the behavior among those who are not experiencing ill health or who are unable or unwilling to see a clinician. Case studies that do not involve death or illness—like the one in the *China Daily* that describes Bao Bao, a perfectly healthy 19-year-old Mongolian girl who has allegedly eaten 1,500 kg of mud since age 7—are rare (2006). Therefore, population-level studies of pica and micronutrient deficiencies are a better measure of both the prevalence of pica and the frequency of association between it and micronutrient deficiencies.

The Pica Literature Database (described in chapter 2) is an example of a more rigorous population-level study of the association between pica and micronutrient deficiency than case studies. There is some reduction in selection bias based on access to medical treatment, and the cultural reports contained in it also span more centuries, geography, and non-ill people than do the individual case reports.

One drawback to the Pica Literature Database is that the measurement of iron deficiency is much less precise in ethnographic reports. There is a reason why micronutrient deficiencies are referred to as "hidden hunger"; it is frequently impossible to tell by mere observation that a person is lacking any requisite micronutrients. However, anemia, in its more severe forms, is one of the easier deficiency conditions to detect by eye. Anemic people appear paler (cf. "Anemia," pp. 58–60, for further discussion). Thus, in the Pica Literature Database, we were able to identify associations with severe anemia when characteristic symptoms such as pallor were described or when anemia or "chlorosis"[3] was "diagnosed" outright by the observer. Such a coarse measurement of anemia means that associations between geophagy with mild anemia would rarely have been detected.

Of the 472 reports in the Pica Literature Database that contained information on the health status, 79 reported information that made it possible to determine if there was a relationship with anemia (*always, sometimes, never*). In more than 77% of reports, anemia was associated with geophagy (fig. 8.1). This was far greater than would be expected under what is called the null hypothesis, or no relationship, in which case we would have expected to see a proportion closer to 33% in each of the three columns.

Still stronger evidence of association is found among the clinic-based observational studies in which a representative population is asked about their pica habits and some measurement of iron status performed. Most of these are cross-sectional observational studies of pregnant women or children in which researchers determined that, indeed, those who engage in pica are more anemic or iron deficient than their non-picaing controls (see Appendix E).

We were able to conduct such analyses in our epidemiological study in Pemba, and observed a very strong association between iron deficiency and pica (Young et al. 2010). After controlling for known confounders (factors

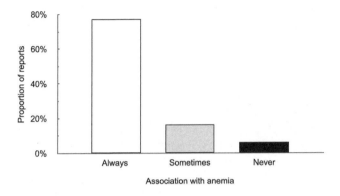

FIGURE 8.1
Frequency with which anemia was associated with geophagy in 79 cultural-level reports in the Pica Literature Database. Anemia was associated with geophagy far more frequently than would be expected if geophagy were equally frequently associated with anemic and non-anemic states.

that could influence both pica behavior and iron status, which in this case included socioeconomic status, gestational age, diet, and infections), the difference in hemoglobin concentration between women who reported no pica and those who reported eating two items was both statistically significant and extremely large from a biological standpoint: 1.1 g/dL.[4]

In summary, there is a very strong relationship between iron deficiency and pica. I would caution you to remember, please, that these are only associations. Based on these data, we cannot even know which came first, the chicken (magpie) or the egg, let alone if they are causally related.

POPULATION-LEVEL ASSOCIATIONS BETWEEN PICA AND ZINC DEFICIENCY

There are far fewer studies of the association between zinc deficiency and pica (Appendix F). Some of the cross-sectional studies of the relationship between anemia and pica (Appendix E) may be a measure of association with zinc deficiency, as zinc is a necessary component of hemoglobin. Despite the smaller number of studies, there are some data to support an association between zinc deficiency and pica. In fact, geophagy was a feature of the first cases of zinc deficiency described in humans. In the early 1960s, Dr. Ananda Prasad described a syndrome in Middle Eastern populations characterized by zinc deficiency, geophagy, iron deficiency anemia, hepatosplenomegaly (enlarged liver and spleen), hypogonadism (underdevelopment of primary and secondary sexual characteristics), and growth retardation (Prasad et al.

1963). Thanks in great part to his work, zinc is now recognized as an essential mineral in human diets (Institute of Medicine 2002).

POPULATION-LEVEL ASSOCIATIONS BETWEEN PICA AND CALCIUM DEFICIENCY

The number of studies that examine the association between iron and zinc deficiencies and pica dwarf those of calcium deficiency. In fact, there has been only one such population-level study, and in it calcium levels were measured rather indirectly. Drs. Andrea Wiley and Sol Katz reviewed ethnographic reports from Africa, and scored each report by the frequency of geophagy (their procedures are described in chapter 2, table 2.1) and by dietary intake (staple foods and dairying practices) (Wiley and Katz 1998). They found that dairying was inversely related to geophagy during pregnancy, i.e., pregnant women were less likely to engage in geophagy in societies in which calcium-rich foods were available. They thus concluded that geophagy during pregnancy could be motivated as a means to increase calcium intake.

Prediction 6. Pica Would Be Associated with Populations with the Highest Micronutrient Requirements

So far, we have looked at case reports and population-level studies of pica to see if associations exist between reported deficiencies and pica. We can also test if associations occur between pica and people with increased micronutrient requirements. In other words, if geophagy is associated with micronutrient deficiencies, we would expect to see it more frequently among those most likely to be experiencing deficiencies.

For many nutrients, including iron, zinc, and calcium, the two populations at greatest risk for deficiencies are pregnant women and children. There are a number of reasons for this, both physiological and social. Pregnant women have a much greater need for nutrients, particularly in the second and third **trimesters** of pregnancy, than do non-pregnant women. This is the time that the fetus begins to require significant amounts of nutrients and the mother's own blood volume needs to expand to be able to feed her rapidly growing bundle of joy.

Young children also grow very quickly and thus require many nutrients for the construction of their quickly expanding little bodies. Furthermore, their small stomachs constrain the amount of food they can ingest, and some nutrient-rich foods, like meats, are not given as frequently as they

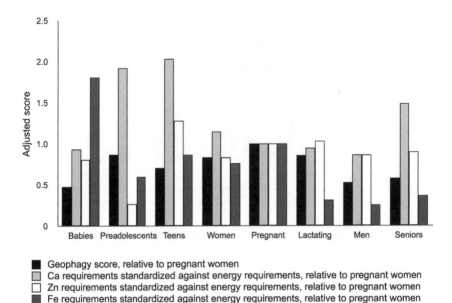

Geophagy score, relative to pregnant women
Ca requirements standardized against energy requirements, relative to pregnant women
Zn requirements standardized against energy requirements, relative to pregnant women
Fe requirements standardized against energy requirements, relative to pregnant women

FIGURE 8.2
Standardized geophagy score and micronutrient requirements (iron, zinc, and calcium), by life stage, relative to pregnant women per Dietary Reference Intake outlined by the Institute of Medicine (2002).

should be, both because of cost and beliefs about their suitability for little ones. In absolute terms, children need smaller amounts of micronutrients than adults do, but relative to their energy intake, they need much more. For example, proportionally, a young child needs three times the amount of iron that an adult man does. For these reasons, absolute requirements are not as indicative of the likelihood of becoming deficient as requirements standardized to energy intake (Institute of Medicine 2002).

The Pica Literature Database permits an examination between geophagy and micronutrient requirements to determine if, indeed, standardized micronutrient requirements predict geophagy (fig. 8.2). You know already that pica occurs frequently among pregnant women and children (cf. chapter 1, p. 16), and so patterns in geophagy initially appear consistent with the micronutrient requirements.

However, the daily reference intakes of micronutrients across various life stage groups do not significantly track the frequency of geophagy (fig. 8.2). In other words, if geophagic soils were consumed to obtain iron, as so many researchers have hypothesized, we would expect infants to

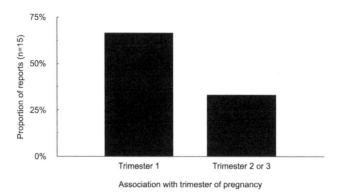

FIGURE 8.3
Timing of geophagy by trimester of pregnancy in the 15 cultural-level reports in the Pica
Literature Database.

ingest earth most frequently, as they have the highest iron requirements.[5]
If zinc supplementation were the impetus for geophagy, it should occur
uniformly across adults, who have similar zinc requirements, but it does
not. And if geophagic soils were consumed for their calcium, as Wiley and
Katz proposed (1998), one would expect preadolescents, adolescents, and
elderly people, who have the highest calcium requirements, to engage in
geophagy most frequently.

Furthermore, if geophagy was a response to micronutrient deficiency,
we would expect earth to be consumed most often in late pregnancy,
when micronutrient requirements are the highest. Women need less iron
in early pregnancy than they do when not pregnant because they are not
losing iron that they typically would through menstruation; in late pregnancy their iron requirements are higher than when not pregnant because
of the needs of the developing fetus (Institute of Medicine 1992). Similarly,
women need less calcium in the early part of pregnancy, since fetal skeletal
growth takes place in mid-pregnancy and most of the calcium is depos-
ited in the fetus in the last trimester (Institute of Medicine 1992). There
is little evidence for additional zinc requirements during pregnancy (Institute of Medicine 1992). However, geophagy does not occur with equal frequency throughout pregnancy (fig. 8.3). It appears most frequently in early
pregnancy, essentially the opposite of what the micronutrient hypothesis
predicts.

Thus, although pica is associated with iron and zinc deficiencies, pica
does not peak during periods of greatest micronutrient requirements.

Prediction 7. Elimination of the Deficiency
Would Cause Pica to Cease

If an iron, zinc, or calcium deficiency caused pica, we would expect that remedying the deficiency would cause the behavior to disappear. In the following sections, I describe the data pertinent to this hypothesis as it pertains to each of the micronutrients.

DOES THE TREATMENT OF IRON DEFICIENCY CAUSE
GEOPHAGY OR AMYLOPHAGY TO END?

Iron has been suggested as a treatment for pica for at least one thousand years. Avicenna, a Persian physician and philosopher who lived in the tenth century, wrote that "pica benefits from iron steeped in fine wine and strained through a Hippocratic sleeve" (quoted in Cooper 1957:10; see also Appendix A).[6] Trotula of Salerno, a female physician in the eleventh century, described geophagy as a treatable problem for pregnant women: "if she desires clay or chalk or coals, let beans cooked with sugar be given to her"(Green 2001); beans are rich in iron. There are plenty of other advocates of iron for the treatment of pica in early medical practice (e.g., Hancock 1831; Michaelis and Boezo 1638).

In modern medicine, iron is also sometimes used to treat pica. Think back to those filing cabinet drawers of case reports that I described earlier in this chapter. In addition to the repetition of associations with iron deficiency and anemia, there is another commonality: treatment of iron deficiency is reported as causing the cessation of pica. In fact, there are scores of case studies of individuals in which the treatment of iron deficiency or anemia coincides with the cessation of pica. Lanzkowsky made a splash in the iron deficiency literature by presenting results from more than one individual: iron dextran injections had caused the cessation of geophagy in twelve South African children (1959). In that same year, Carlander described how, of his approximately 100 patients with pica (characteristics not specified besides "mostly women"), all of them had iron deficiency and most, but not all, were anemic (Carlander 1959). Within approximately two weeks of treatment with iron, their pica disappeared.

After reading a few dozen descriptions of individual case studies, it becomes easy to believe that the correction of anemia can cure pica. But there are many reasons to be skeptical of such a conclusion based on these data. The roles played by medical attention and advice, other treatments administered, the placebo effect of these interventions, and the absence of controls all make causal inferences untenable. We need data from more rigorous studies to draw conclusions.

Unfortunately, there are only a few experimental studies of the effects of micronutrient supplements on pica. Four of the studies in which participants were given either iron or a control involved children, either in the United States (Gutelius et al. 1962), South Africa (McDonald and Marshall 1964), India (Mohan et al. 1968), or Zambia (Nchito et al. 2004); one involved pregnant women in the United States (Rogers 1972). In U.S. studies of children and pregnant women, there were no significant differences in pica behavior by treatment received, i.e., iron supplementation did not cause pica to cease. The studies in South Africa and India were sufficiently flawed in design, execution, and analysis to be inconclusive. The most sophisticated study of the effect of iron supplementation on pica behavior took place among 402 Zambian schoolchildren (Nchito et al. 2004). In this randomized, controlled trial of micronutrient supplementation and geophagy, neither daily administration of iron (for ten months) nor a multivitamin without iron significantly reduced geophageous behavior.

Basically, available data do not support that remedying iron deficiency causes a decrease in geophagy or amylophagy.

DOES THE TREATMENT OF IRON DEFICIENCY CAUSE PAGOPHAGY TO END?

In the course of my research on pica, I have had a number of confessional-type conversations in which pediatricians, professors, and nurses have told me how they inexplicably took to crunching large quantities of ice, only to desist after they were treated for iron deficiency that they had not been aware of. Individual cases are, as you know by now, the weakest form of evidence, and conclusions based on these data alone are very weak. As counterintuitive as it may seem, however, the little experimental evidence that is available seems to provide some support for iron deficiency causing pagophagy. Caution must be used, however, since there are only two such studies.

In 1969, Coltman conducted a single-blind study of seven iron-deficient adult women patients at a U.S. airforce base (1969; see also fig. 8.4). Their baseline weekly ice consumption was quantified, and then participants were given intramuscular injections of saline. Their ice consumption was not statistically significantly different. The following week, they were given intramuscular injections of iron. Ice consumption diminished rapidly, but did not disappear completely (the authors attributed this to an inadequate dose of iron). The strongest evidence in support of iron deficiency causing pica comes from a study in which anemic rats consumed a significantly

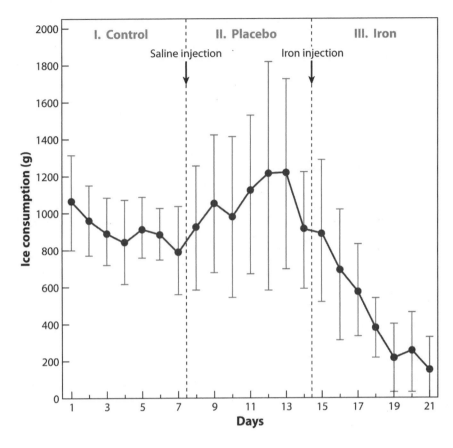

FIGURE 8.4
Mean ±1 standard deviation of the daily ice consumption of 7 pagophagists during the
3 phases of Coltman's single-blind study (1969): (I) The Control phase represents the
baseline, with no intervention; (II) in the Placebo phase, participants received intramuscular
injections of 5 cc of saline; and (III) the Iron phase shows the week during which participants
received intramuscular injections of 5 cc of iron dextran. Redrawn from Coltman (1969);
reprinted by permission of *Annual Reviews*.

greater proportion of their daily water in the form of ice than non-anemic
controls (Woods and Weisinger 1970). Anemic rats chose to consume 96%
of their water in the form of ice; non-anemic controls consumed only 45%
as ice. Recovery from anemia reduced pagophagy.

In summary, the two intervention studies that have examined if the correction of iron deficiency caused the cessation of ice-eating suggest that correction may sometimes cause pagophagy to disappear, but the extremely
small sample size and limited number of studies clearly indicate that more

work is needed. It would be particularly useful to elucidate a mechanism by which this may occur.

DOES THE TREATMENT OF ZINC DEFICIENCY CAUSE PICA TO END?

There have been only three studies of the effects of zinc supplementation on human pica behavior. Two were conducted among children in India (Bhalla et al. 1983) and China (Chen et al. 1985); one was conducted among mentally retarded adults in the United States (Lofts et al. 1990). Pica behavior dramatically decreased after zinc was given to the children. In the study among adults, after zinc was given, the average number of pica incidents per person fell from 23 to 4.3 incidents over a two-week period.

The studies were not ideal. For example, none of them used controls, nor was there any indication of other messages given to participants, e.g., verbal encouragement to not eat earth. Furthermore, neither of the studies in children actually measured changes in zinc status; therefore we can't know if any changes in pica behavior were even associated with changes in zinc levels.

In short, in all of these studies the cessation of pica has been observed after the administration of zinc, but many factors were altered in addition to zinc concentrations, so that it is not possible to state that the return to normal zinc values was the causal factor of the disappearance of pica. Sufficient data are simply not currently available to permit definitive conclusions about the efficacy of zinc treatment in causing the cessation of pica.

DOES THE TREATMENT OF CALCIUM DEFICIENCY CAUSE PICA TO END?

There are almost no experimental data with which to test the hypothesis that remedying calcium deficiency causes the cessation of pica. In fact, only one small study has investigated the effects of calcium, in a mixture with other vitamins and minerals, on pica behavior (Gutelius et al. 1963). In this study, twelve U.S. children with pica were given a multivitamin and mineral supplement (that contained no iron) daily for six to seven weeks; twelve other children with pica were given placebos. After seven weeks of treatment, five had pica in each group; three to thirteen months after treatment ended, three in each group had pica. In sum, neither calcium nor the other micronutrients in the supplement affected pica behavior. To date, this is the only experimental evidence to test the calcium hypothesis.

All in all, experimental evidence does not indicate that the treatment of micronutrient deficiencies reduces non-ice picas; it may have some impact on the reduction of pagophagy.

Prediction 8. Pica Substances Would Provide Micronutrients in Which the Consumer is Deficient

Piglets with access to exposed earth do not become anemic (Hyslop 1977). Cattle gnaw on bones when their diet is deficient in phosphorous, thereby increasing their phosphorous levels (Foster 1927; Green 1925). In a recent study, when sheep were made zinc-deficient, they began to gnaw into the plaster walls around their pen, which, as it turned out, were high in zinc (Kendall and Telfer 2000). These anecdotes thus beg the question—if livestock can obtain nutrients by eating items they would not normally eat, can humans? If pica is an adaptive response to micronutrient deficiencies, we can expect pica materials to contain bioavailable iron, zinc, and/or calcium. Each of these micronutrients will be examined in turn, below.

HOW ABOUT THAT IRON?

Some pica substances clearly contain very little iron, e.g., uncooked rice, cornstarch, and chalk. The micronutrient content of other pica items is less obvious, particularly that of earth.

One source of data on iron content in geophagic soils comes from the Pica Literature Database. The color of the soils consumed was described in 160 reports. Geophagic samples ranged in color from bright white to light yellow, orange, red, red-brown, purple, dark gray, black, blue, and light green. Red hues, indicative of iron, were reported in 44% of the 160 descriptions of geophagic soils. Interestingly, when there was a choice between red and other colors of clay, the non-red clays were typically preferred.[7] Although data on iron content of the soils in the Pica Literature Database is very imprecise, it offers some of the broadest range of information we have on physical properties of geophagic soils.

Fortunately, we have better data than mere color descriptions to evaluate this prediction. There have been dozens of chemical analyses of geophagic soils, although these data are less useful than one would expect. Why? A total acid digest is the typical analysis performed on geophagic soils in the last two hundred years, and many have indicated that iron or zinc is present in geophagic samples (e.g., Cotting 1836). Unfortunately, we cannot use any of these data to conclude if humans can obtain iron from soil. Why not? In total acid digests, substances are completely dissolved in a strongly acidic solution, and their elemental composition is then calculated. This almost certainly overestimates the nutrient content (Wilson 2003).

When we digest food, the food is first processed in the very acidic environment of our stomach, which is similar to (although less intense than) the total acid digest described above. However, in the next phase of digestion, the contents of the stomach move to the intestine, where the pH is more neutral (pH approximately 7). It is here where the bulk of iron absorption takes place. At this higher (less acidic) pH, iron is not very soluble. Thus, equating the total elemental composition with the amounts that are bioavailable leads to overestimation. This means that a number of scientists have concluded that iron is available from geophagic samples when, in fact, they have not performed tests that permit such a conclusion.

For example, Dr. John Hunter stated that he examined the bioavailability of iron in geophagic clays from Belize (Hunter and de Kleine 1984), Ghana (Hunter 1973), and Sierra Leone (Hunter 1984), but the method[8] he and his collaborators used ignores much of the biochemistry of the alimentary canal—most critically, the pH of the intestine. Nevertheless, Hunter concluded that "until they are superseded in Africa by cheap and easily obtainable pharmaceutical products, [geophagic soils] will continue to offer rough-and-ready but valuable and wide-ranging, mineral supplementation" (Hunter 1973). Dr. William Mahaney, who has published widely on geophagy, has also overlooked alimentary biochemistry in his and his research group's many otherwise excellent analyses of geophagic materials (e.g., Aufreiter et al. 2001; Krishnamani and Mahaney 2000; Mahaney et al. 2000; Mahaney et al. 2005). Thus, their conclusions about high iron concentrations in soils (Mahaney et al. 2000; Mahaney, et al. 2005) must be questioned. A greater familiarity with gut pH would have likely prevented a number of other scientists (Bolton et al. 1998; Ferrell 2008; Georgette and Francis 2003; Gilardi et al. 1999; Hladik and Gueguen 1974; Johns and Duquette 1991a) from similarly conflating total elemental composition with bioavailability.

HOW ABOUT THAT *BIOAVAILABLE* IRON?

The consideration of bioavailability is rare; only five studies in which geophagic earth was analyzed have considered intestinal biochemistry in their analyses. Two studies have used the physiologically based extraction test (based on Ruby et al. 1996) to study Ugandan (Smith et al. 2000) and Indian geophagic soils (Abrahams et al. 2006). This in vitro (i.e., in glassware, not in a living organism) technique is a closer approximation to the human digestive system than the total acid digests, as the process involves a phase that mimics the pH and digestive enzymes in the gut. As expected, the availability of many elements under gut conditions was far lower than with total elemental analyses, e.g., < 5% of total iron and even less zinc was bioavailable across all samples in these two studies. A third study in which intestinal conditions were attempted to be replicated was conducted by Dreyer and colleagues on a black and a red sample of South African geophagic soils (2004). Neither substance provided bioavailable iron or zinc, and one could possibly provide calcium and magnesium.

Kikouama and colleagues investigated trace elements released by six West African geophagic clays under either oral, gastric, or intestinal conditions (samples were not passed through each stage consecutively (2008). They found the availability of both ferric and ferrous Fe to be lowest under intestinal pH, but did not calculate potential Fe contribution, likely because of the absence of information on amount of earth consumed.

Hooda and collaborators (2004) conducted the most sophisticated study of bioavailability by looking at the nutrients that geophagic materials could contribute in vitro *as well as* at their capacity to bind nutrients in suspension, thus rendering them unavailable. Their results indicated that the five geophagic samples from around the world significantly *reduced* the availability of iron and zinc in suspension, suggesting that soils do not contribute micronutrients and are likely to bind the iron and zinc available in ingested foods (fig. 8.5).

In brief, the idea that humans are consuming earth as a response to iron deficiency is an attractive theory because of its simplicity, but no data exist that suggest that pica substances contain substantial quantities of bioavailable iron and can therefore improve low iron status.

BIOAVAILABILITY OF ZINC

Data on the presence and bioavailability of zinc in geophagic earth are scantier still. In 1970, Smith and Halsted conducted the only in vivo study (study done in living organisms) of the micronutrient bioavailability of geophagic soils. They concluded that modified[9] geophagic soil from Iran could contribute dietary zinc to rats (Smith and Halsted 1970). Their findings are in contrast to the data on bioavailability from in vitro analyses

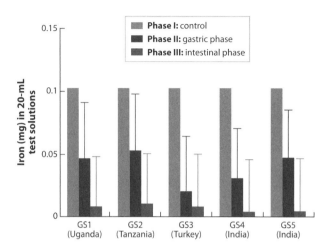

FIGURE 8.5
The effect of geophagy simulation on potentially bioavailable iron in 5 earth samples in a solution of iron (redrawn from Hooda et al. 2004). A change in iron content of the control solution following the gastric (phase 1) and intestinal (phase 2) simulations signifies a potential loss/gain in its bioavailability. Error bars on phase 1 and phase 2 represent least significant difference (LSD) when a nutrient in the control solution was compared with that following phase-1 and phase-2 simulation, respectively, for soil ingestion. Reprinted by permission of *Annual Reviews*.

of unmodified geophagic soils discussed above, in which little zinc was available (Smith and Halsted 1970; Abrahams et al. 2006; Dreyer et al. 2004) and that some geophagic soils bound dietary zinc, rendering it unavailable (Hooda et al. 2004). These differences could be due to the fact that the removal of calcium affected zinc bioavailability, or that, as Hooda and colleagues (2004) pointed out, different soils can offer different micronutrients.

The bioavailability of zinc in other pica substances (e.g., freezer frost from older freezers with zinc linings and raw starches) has not been analyzed and would certainly be useful for testing this hypothesis. At present, there is insufficient evidence to determine the bioavailability of zinc in pica substances.

BIOAVAILABILITY OF CALCIUM

There is little discussion of the potential for pica substances to provide calcium, although calcium deficiency seems to be the most biologically plausible. A number of pica substances such as chalk, ground shells, and plaster are rich in calcium, and calcium is much more readily absorbed by the body than is iron or zinc. That said, when Wiley and Katz reviewed estimates of bioavailability of fifteen geophagic soils, they determined that only three could provide more than 10% of the recommended daily allowance for calcium (Wiley and Katz 1998). Hooda and coworkers did, however, suggest that geophagic substances provide bioavailable calcium (Hooda et al. 2004). Currently, there is insufficient evidence to test this hypothesis.

A MALADAPTIVE RESPONSE?

Most scientists have suggested that pica is an adaptive response to a micronutrient deficiency, i.e., pica is a strategy for obtaining the missing nutrient. An alternative explanation of the association between pica and micronutrient deficiencies is that pica is a response to a micronutrient deficiency, but a nonadaptive one, i.e., it does not increase micronutrient status. Under this hypothesis, pica is considered an aberrant epiphenomenon; the resultant cravings are not for the substances that will remedy the deficiency, they are simply a product of a malfunctioning brain.

How might this work? Suggested mechanisms have been rather vague. Youdim and Iancu attribute abnormal cravings to iron and zinc deficiencies in "key appetite-regulating brain enzymes" (1977). Von Bonsdorff posits that the iron-rich hypothalamus, responsible for regulating appetite, might not function properly in the absence of sufficient iron, and thus cause pica (1977). E. R. Eichner speculates that the "cells lining the mouth run out of iron and send an alarm signal to the brain" (quoted in Anderson 2005), but he was unable to specify which cells these might be (personal communication, 9/30/03). More plausible research suggests that taste sensitivity may be altered by zinc deficiency (Chisholm and Martin 1981; Prasad 1996); this in turn could cause non-food substances to have an appealing taste.

A nonadaptive explanation of pica is difficult to embrace for a number of reasons. For one, the persistence of pica in the animal kingdom suggests that there is an adaptive benefit. Second, patterns in pica behavior point to other ways in which pica may contribute to fitness (cf. chapter 9).

Thus, for the present, we must conclude that pica substances provide little in the way of the micronutrients whose deficiencies they are associated with, both in absolute terms as well as when bioavailability is considered.

Could Pica *Cause* a Micronutrient Deficiency?

Despite the strong association between pica and micronutrient deficiencies (Prediction 5), treatment of the deficiency does not cause the cessation of pica (Prediction 7), nor do pica substances provide much in the way of iron, zinc, or calcium (Prediction 8). So, how to explain the association between pica and micronutrient deficiencies?

One possibility is that there is no causal relationship.[10] Another possibility is that pica, rather than remedying micronutrient deficiencies, exacerbates them. Pica could cause a micronutrient deficiency in three ways: by replacing iron-rich foods with non-nutritive items, by causing geohelminth infections that result in blood loss or poor micronutrient absorption, or by binding with dietary micronutrients, rendering them unusable.

The replacement mechanism (Keith et al. 1968) is unlikely; pica substances tend to be eaten in addition to the foods that would normally be consumed, not in place of them (Cooksey 1995; Edwards et al. 1959). Soil has been used instead of food only when food is unavailable (cf. chapter 7).

Several facts suggest that geohelminth infection also cannot explain the strong association between pica and micronutrient deficiencies. Most earths are collected from areas unlikely to be contaminated with geohelminths, and many earths are heated prior to consumption which would kill the geohelminths (Vermeer and Frate 1979; Young et al. 2007; also, see "Geohelminths" in chapter 5). Furthermore, other pica substances such as ice and cornstarch are unlikely to be vectors for geohelminth infection, and anemia is associated with pica even in areas where geohelminth infections are rare.

The third mechanism by which pica may cause a micronutrient deficiency is through the inhibition of micronutrient absorption. This could occur if substances either bind micronutrients in ingested food or decrease the permeability of the mucin layer in the intestine, which is where much micronutrient absorption happens. Given the fact that many clays have both high surface-to-volume ratio and high cation exchange capacity (see "The Amazing Properties of Clays" in chapter 3), this explanation is the most plausible.

Studies of Inhibition of Iron Absorption by Pica Substances

A handful of small studies have investigated the effect of pica substances on iron absorption using **radio-labeled iron**. Earth has been the primary substance investigated, but absorption studies have also been conducted using starch and ash.

There have been a number of studies of the effects of geographic earth on iron absorption. All three studies of Turkish geophagic clay have shown that it inhibits iron absorption in humans (Arcasoy et al. 1978; Cavdar and Arcasoy 1972; Minnich et al. 1968). Among adults with normal iron status, 27% of iron (in the form of $FeSO_4$) was absorbed in the absence of clay, while only 2% was absorbed when iron was ingested five minutes after eating clay (Cavdar and Arcasoy 1972). Among iron-deficient adults (who tend to up-regulate their iron metabolism and can thereby absorb more iron than iron-replete individuals), 46% of iron was absorbed when clay had not been ingested, compared to only 6% when it had been (Cavdar and Arcasoy 1972). Similar differences were seen when **heme iron** (iron that has already been integrated into hemoglobin) was ingested with and without Turkish clay (Cavdar and Arcasoy 1972). In South Africa, iron absorption was also greatly decreased when earth was eaten prior to the ingestion of iron (mean 17.4% without earth vs. 5% with earth) (Sayers et al. 1974). Results from studies of U.S. geophagic soils indicated that some, but not all, inhibited iron absorption. Inhibited iron absorption was seen with geophagic clays from Mississippi and Georgia, but not New Mexico (Cavdar and Arcasoy 1972). Two popular Texas geophagic clays were found to have little impact on iron absorption (Talkington et al. 1970).

Three studies of the effects of starch on iron absorption have been conducted. Blum and colleagues determined that starch consumption caused iron absorption to be reduced from 93% to 40% (Blum et al. 1968). In contrast, in Talkington and colleagues' work, iron absorption was not significantly different in the presence of 60 g of starch (Talkington et al. 1970). In 1976, Thomas and coauthors conducted the most rigorous study of the capacity of laundry starch to bind both inorganic ($FeSO_4$) and heme iron (Thomas et al. 1976). In incubating flasks, laundry starch bound 19 to 80% of the available $FeSO_4$ and 34 to 68% of the available heme iron; maximal binding occurred at pH 7.0, the pH of the intestine. In both anemic and non-anemic rats, administration of a suspension of laundry starch prior to the ingestion of either type of iron caused significantly lower absorption of iron compared to those given the saline control solution. However, when laundry starch was administered simultaneously with or after ingestion of iron, iron absorption was not reduced. These data indicate that laundry starch can bind appreciable quantities of iron in vitro and in vivo.

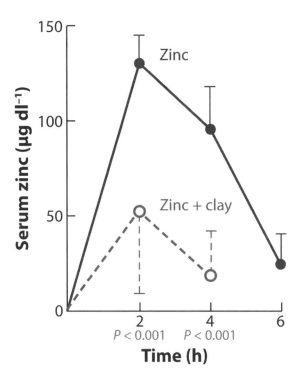

FIGURE 8.6
Oral zinc absorption (mean ± 1 SD) with and without prior ingestion of 5 g of Turkish geophagic clay (n = 17). Redrawn from Cavdar and colleagues (1983); reprinted by permission of *Annual Reviews*.

In the sole study of iron absorption and ash, iron absorption in the presence of ash was inhibited (14.5% vs. 9.6%) (Sayers et al. 1974).

Studies of Inhibition of Zinc Absorption by Geophagic Earth

The effects of clay on zinc absorption were studied among seventeen Turkish children and adults with iron deficiency anemia (Arcasoy et al. 1978); twelve were geophagists, five were not. Zinc was orally administered and serum zinc was measured at baseline, two, four, and six hours after the test dose. All patients with geophagy demonstrated impaired zinc absorption. Another study of zinc absorption among seventeen non-geophagists again showed that zinc consumed with 5 g of clay impeded zinc absorption (Cavdar et al. 1983; see also fig. 8.6). The authors suggested that earth might bind not just with dietary zinc but also with endogenous zinc released from the pancreas.

Studies of Inhibition of Potassium Absorption by Geophagic Earth

Pica substances may bind **cations** other than iron, zinc, and calcium. Potassium is a good example. There have been a number of reports of clay-induced hypokalemia (low potassium) (e.g., Dreyer et al. 2004; Gonzalez et al. 1982; Severance et al. 1988). Biochemical analyses of geophagic samples offer mechanistic support. Dreyer and colleagues showed that potassium is absorbed by a black soil ingested in South Africa (Dreyer et al. 2004). Gonzalez and coworkers examined clay that seemed to be causing hypokalemia in a patient in Wilmington, North Carolina, and revealed that, indeed, under in vitro conditions, the addition of clay bound approximately 30% of potassium in solution (Gonzalez et al. 1982). Potassium-binding capacities were also identified in clay from a geophagist in Greenville, North Carolina (Severance et al. 1988).

Based on these small micronutrient absorption studies, we can conclude that *some* pica substances are able to interfere with the absorption of some micronutrients. Differences in observed effects of pica on micronutrient absorption may be attributable to varying physical and chemical properties of the pica substances (e.g., cation exchange capacity), variation in time elapsed between ingestion of the pica substance and micronutrient of interest, or unmeasured changes in the subjects' own iron metabolism across time.

In sum, although there is an association between iron and zinc deficiencies and pica (Prediction 5), there is evidence that contradicts the supplementation hypothesis. For one, pica does not track micronutrient needs through the life span or within pregnancy. Second, micronutrient supplementation has not been proven to cause the cessation of non-ice picas (Prediction 7). In the two studies of iron supplementation and pagophagy, iron supplementation has shown some promise in reducing ice consumption, but more thorough research is needed to confirm this. If pica was an adaptive response to micronutrient deficiency, the irregular presence of micronutrients and their probable low bioavailability make it unlikely that pica substances can function as micronutrient supplements (Prediction 8). All in all, existing data do not lend much support to the supplementation hypothesis. In fact, the opposite of supplementation may be happening; pica substances may be causing micronutrient deficiencies. Experimental evidence supports the idea that some pica substances interfere with the absorption of micronutrients and can thus contribute to deficiencies.

But why would animals and humans eat non-food substances if they only caused a negative outcome, i.e., micronutrient deficiencies?[11] Perhaps the consequences of pica are not only negative; we still have one more adaptive hypothesis to explore.

CHAPTER NINE

Pica to Protect and Detoxify

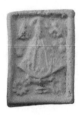 THE FINAL adaptive hypothesis is the protection-detoxification hypothesis. Under this hypothesis, pica is a protective behavior, one that shields us from the harmful items we ingest. This mechanism is dramatically illustrated by the plight of an English prisoner sentenced to death in 1581 for his thieving ways:

> One called Wendel Thumblardt was by our Lieutenant of Langenburg for certaine fellonies imprisoned, who being examined by our Justices confessed himself guilty of a great number of robberies: And therefore brought to the barre was condemned to bee hanged. Being yet deteined in prison, and coming to his eare that there was such a medicine, so soveraigne against sundrie sicknesses, and the most deadly poisons, has made humble request as well by his parents, as by other his friends, of which there were present no small number, desiring for the mercie of God, and respect of his poor life, that being thus condemned, hee might have given unto him the most deadly poison that might be devised, whereby a perfit triall might bee had of the worthines of this medicinable earth. (quoted in Thompson 1914:436)

On the appointed day, nobility and commoners assembled to see this confessed-thief-cum-lab rat given a dram and a half of "Mercurie Sublimate, mingled with Conserve of Roses." Mercury poisoning is excruciating; it corrodes the mucus membranes and stomach lining and induces severe nausea, abdominal pain, diarrhea, renal damage, and death. And the amount of mercury sublimate our plundering Wendel swallowed was at least three times the amount needed to kill an average-size man (Root-Bernstein and Root-Bernstein 1997:60).

Immediately after he drank the mercury, he drank wine in which approximately 4 grams of terra sigillata (cf. chapter 3) had been dissolved. After much anguish, "the poison did extremely torment and vexe him," the terra sigillata prevailed: Wendel survived. He was released from the courts and delivered to his parents.

This story vividly demonstrates the ability of clay to shield us from harm, which is, of course, a property integral to the protection-detoxification hypothesis. Before delving into the predictions of this hypothesis (see Appendix G), I will present some relevant background information, namely what pica may be protecting us from, and the mechanisms by which it may occur.

Toxins and Pathogens

It may at first be surprising to you that plants are a major source of toxins. However, since plants cannot protect themselves by running away from predators, their best strategy for avoiding being grazed upon is to make themselves less appetizing. Thorns and sticky resins are easily detectable examples of plant defense tactics, but they have other, nonmechanical strategies. Many plants produce toxic chemicals, such as alkaloids, tannins, saponins, phenolics, and terpenes, to protect themselves from both the insects and larger animals who want to eat them, as well as smaller microbes that may cause them disease. Such compounds are called **secondary compounds** or secondary metabolites—"secondary" because these chemicals are not involved in the normal growth, development, or reproduction of the organism.[1]

Plants are not the only organisms to produce harmful chemicals: molds and bacteria do, too. Fungi produce mycotoxins, such as the highly carcinogenic aflatoxin, for the express purpose of persuading vertebrates like us to leave food alone once they have staked a claim (Barlow 2000). Some bacteria produce enterotoxins, poisons that help them to efficiently colonize the gut. We may also encounter harmful chemical compounds formed through various high-temperature food preparation techniques, especially frying and grilling (Skog 1993).

All of these chemical compounds produced by plants and pathogens can cause gastrointestinal distress, dizziness, and muscle pains. In sufficient quantities they can be teratogenic (harm fetuses), mutagenic (cause mutations in cells), carcinogenic (cause cancer), or downright lethal (Hui et al. 2001b). We thus need to be protected from the harmful effects of toxins; pica substances may do just that.

The second type of injurious items that pica may protect us from are food and waterborne pathogens. These include harmful bacteria like those that cause nonspecific diarrhea (e.g., *Escherichia coli, Staphylococcus aureus*) as well as those that cause more acute, scarier infections including botulism, salmonella, and listeriosis. Bigger-than-bacteria pathogens that are best steered clear from include amoebas, roundworms, and flatworms. All of these pathogens can do terrible things to our bodies either directly (e.g., by causing unnecessary blood loss or poor nutrient absorption) or through the release of enterotoxins. Infections with most of these multisyllabic evildoers usually involve a range of symptoms associated with gastrointestinal distress, from nausea, to vomiting, to acute and copious diarrhea.

Besides just being unpleasant, the consequences of infections by food and waterborne pathogens can be very dangerous. Let's take just one example: diarrhea. During episodes of diarrhea, food and water is evacuated before it is fully processed; this means that diarrhea robs us of hard-earned nutrients and calories before they can be metabolized. Our intestinal lining also becomes inflamed, further reducing absorption. On top of all that, the inflammatory response that we mount to fight off the infection causes our metabolism to increase, which means that we burn calories faster. Thus, cruelly, even as we take in fewer calories, we expend more than usual. In a well-nourished person, diarrhea is frequently little more than a nuisance, but for marginally healthy people, it can be deadly. Indeed, it is lethal for far too many individuals every year. It is responsible for the deaths of approximately 2,000,000 children annually. That's 238 children every hour.

The Protective Capacity of Clays

Clays can offer protection from harmful toxins and pathogens by reinforcing the intestinal wall (fig. 9.1). Our intestines are lined with a nice slippery layer of mucus that protects the epithelial cells, the intestinal cells that come into the most contact with everything you swallow. This mucus is an important physical and chemical shield for the rest of the body; it is at this juncture that most food and waterborne pathogens enter our bloodstream.

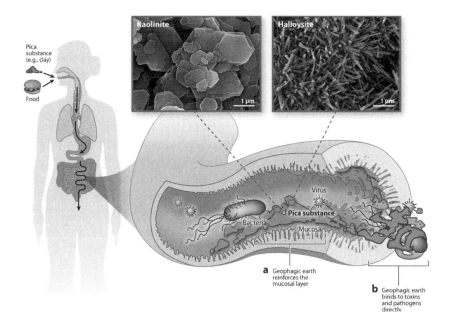

FIGURE 9.1
Geophagic earth may protect against toxins and pathogens by (a) strengthening the mucosal layer by binding with mucin and/or stimulating mucin production, thereby reducing the permeability of the gut wall and (b) binding to toxins and pathogens directly, thereby rendering them unabsorbable by the gut. Scanning electron microscope photo insets kindly provided by Evelyne Delbos of the Macaulay Institute. Illustration by Fiona R. Martin. Reprinted by permission from *Annual Review of Nutrition*.

But the mucosal layer is regularly eroded by acidic foods such as Tabasco sauce and bourbon (two of my favorite aggressors), stomach acid, and bacterial or viral pathogens. When this happens, it's easier for harmful chemicals and pathogens to enter our bloodstream. Clays, therefore, could offer protection by reinforcing the mucosal layer.

Both smectite (Gonzalez et al. 2004) and palygorskite (More et al. 1987) have been demonstrated to be able to fortify the intestinal barrier by cross-linking with molecules in mucus. Smectite has even been shown to *cause* increased mucin production (Gonzalez et al. 2004). It is possible that other clays could work similarly to reinforce the mucin layer, although no others have been studied.

You will recall from chapter 3 ("What Is a Clay?") that clays are good at adsorbing positively charged molecules' cations (the "peanut butter") on their negatively charged layers (the "bread"). This adsorption capacity means that clays can offer an organism protection by binding toxins and pathogens to them before they can even reach the gut wall (fig. 9.1). In other words, clay can deactivate toxins not by destroying them, but by grabbing them before they can be digested, adsorbing them into some of that space in its crystal structure. Unwanted chemicals and pathogens trapped in clays then move out of the body with other solid waste.

There is ample experimental evidence of the ability of clays to bind all kinds of plant toxins, viruses, fungi, and bacteria (Young 2010).[2] Some of the most extensive studies on the protective activity of clay have been done in rats, who are not able to rid themselves of toxins by throwing up. They will eat kaolin when exposed to nausea-inducing conditions and success- fully reduce poison-related sickness and death (Liu et al. 2005; Madden 1998; Mccaffrey 1985; Mitchell et al. 1976; Takeda et al. 1993), just like Wendel did in 1581.

With this brief background on how protection and detoxification of tox- ins and pathogens may occur, let's move to the predictions of this hypoth- esis. If pica is a protective or detoxifying practice, we would expect:

Prediction 9. Pica substances would shield us from the harmful effects of toxins and pathogens.

Prediction 10. Pica would occur more frequently during exposure to tox- ins and pathogens.

Prediction 11. Pica would occur more frequently when people are vulner- able to the harmful effects of toxins and pathogens.

Testing the Protection Hypothesis

Prediction 9. Pica Substances Would Shield Us from the Harmful Effects of Toxins and Pathogens

GEOPHAGIC EARTH

Under the protection-detoxification hypothesis, pica substances should, well, protect us. We already know that clays are excellent at binding mol- ecules. And we know that most geophagic earths contain a high proportion of clay (cf. chapter 1, p. 5). Of the 99 geophagic earths in the Pica Literature Database whose physical characteristics were described, 98 had claylike properties. Analyses of 12 geophagic soil samples from Pemba indicated the presence of the clay mineral group kaolin in all of them (Young et al. 2010b).

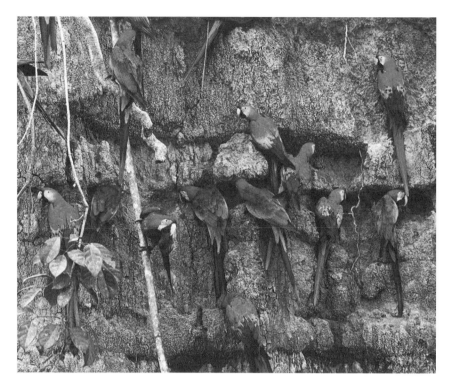

FIGURE 9.2
Scarlet and Red-and-Green Macaws in Manu, Peru, engaged in geophagy. Many species of parrots can be found in large numbers in sites with abundant clay, called clay licks. Parrots tend to congregate at one soil band, ignoring earth one meter above and below. Although the most famous parrot clay licks are in Peru, they have also been discovered throughout Latin America, central Africa, and Papua New Guinea. Photo © generously provided courtesy of World Parrot Trust (www.parrots.org).

Although we know that clays are excellent detoxifiers, there have been only two experiments about the detoxifying and protective capacities of earths that are actually eaten; the rest of the studies have used purified clays. This dearth of data is mostly due to the fact that this is the newest of the hypotheses about pica; there hasn't been enough time to test it fully.[3]

The first such experiment was conducted by Dr. Timothy Johns, a professor of nutrition at McGill University, together with his colleague Dr. Martin Duquette (1991a). They tested the capacity of 18 different samples of geophagic earths from California, Italy, a number of African countries, and clay found at the site of *Homo habilis* (cf. chapter 1, p. 17) to bind tannic acid. Not only did all samples contain kaolinite and/or smectite, all clays were able to bind plant secondary compounds under in vitro conditions.

Dr. James Gilardi, a behavioral ecologist, together with colleagues at the University of California, Davis, conducted an incredibly rigorous, in-depth study of the potential detoxifying effects of earth consumed by Amazonian parrots (1999; see also fig. 9.2).[4] To do this, they administered a solution of clay and quinidine sulfate (a plant toxin) to four parrots using a feeding tube, and a solution of water (no clay) and quinidine to the other four. They sampled blood from all parrots at one, two, and three hours postdose. Two weeks later, they reversed which four parrots got the toxins. Circulating quinidine levels in parrots dosed with clay were approximately 60% lower than their buddies who got the control. In short, geophagic clay prevented these birds from absorbing plant toxins.

CHARCOAL

Charcoal is an extremely powerful adsorbent, especially in its activated form. **Activated charcoal** is basically regular charcoal that has been processed with steam at *very* high temperatures. This processing makes it extremely porous, which means it has a very large surface area. One teaspoon of activated carbon has a surface area the size of a football field, just as some clays do. Because a large surface area makes it extremely adsorptive, activated charcoal is used in all kinds of industrial applications (Cooney 1995). It does the binding in your Brita water filter; it filters the air in gas masks and in spacesuit Primary Life Support Systems. Charcoal traps mercury emissions from coal-fired power stations and medical incinerators. And charcoal is integral to the Lincoln County Process, a technique for filtering Tennessee whiskey through a column of charcoal chips before it goes into casks for aging.

There are also a number of medical uses for activated charcoal (Cooney 1995). It is the treatment of choice for the ingestion of many poisons by humans and animals. Poison Control Centers recommend all homes with small children have activated charcoal on hand. In Europe, it is commonly used to treat diarrhea, where it is sold in an over-the-counter preparation called NORIT.

Laboratory experiments indicate that activated charcoal is frequently as effective as clay as a detoxifier. Both montmorillonite, a type of clay, and activated charcoal were successfully used in hemoperfusion[5] of laboratory animals poisoned with paraquat, a highly toxic weed killer (Lotan et al. 1983). Giving activated charcoal and/or clay to 24 fasting female laboratory rabbits prevented them from dying from a lethal dose of paraquat; the six who did not have the protection of clay or charcoal all died (Okonek et al. 1982). And experimental analyses of charcoal consumed by colobus monkeys indicated it was able to detoxify harmful plant secondary compounds (Cooney and Struhsaker 1997; Struhsaker et al. 1997), as described below.

STARCH

Like clay and charcoal, raw starch is good at absorbing and binding. This binding capacity motivates the inclusion of a few grains of rice in salt shakers (to absorb moisture, preventing the salt from caking), advice to submerge a sodden iPhone in a bowl of uncooked rice to dry it out, and the use of a variety of starches in pressing clothes (cf. chapter 1). But starches have many other unsung industrial accomplishments (Ellis et al. 1998). In the medical world, cornstarch is used in wound dressings and orally administered in a solution of water to treat iodine poisoning. Outside of hospitals, it is found in face powders, batteries, fuel filters, disposable diapers, and baby powders. Papermaking is the largest non-food application for starch; every year, 3.5 million pounds of starch are used in the manufacture of paper in North America alone. In papermaking, starches have two functions. Cationic starches (remember the cation exchange capacity of clays?) are mixed with wet paper pulp. They bind tightly with cellulose, the woody pulp, which is negatively charged; this increases the strength of paper. Starches are used again after the paper has dried. A starch coating on paper acts as a sizing (that is, it curbs the bleeding of ink), binding it to the surface of the paper where it was applied. Because of these handy-dandy uses of starch in papermaking, a typical sheet of copy paper can contain as much as 8% starch. Indeed, if you are reading this book on paper, the paper on which it is printed, Thomson-Shore's #50 Nature's Natural, contains cornstarch.

With your burgeoning knowledge of the physical properties of pica substances, it should be no surprise to learn that once they cross your lips, these items are still good at binding. Ingesting clay, starch, charcoal, and/or magnesium trisilicate (a common antacid) at the same time you take medicines has repeatedly been shown to inhibit their effectiveness. Antibiotics (Khalil et al. 1976; Ofoefule and Okonta 1999), heart medicines (Brown and Juhl 1976), and antimalarials (McElnay et al. 1982) have also been demonstrated to be bound by these non-food items. In one in vitro experiment, researchers studied the capacity of charcoal, clay, starch (derived from a Nigerian tuber called *tacca*), and magnesium trisilicate, to bind with

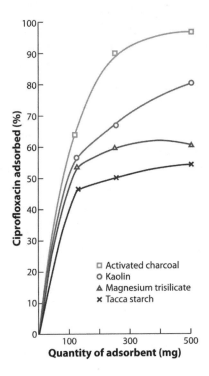

FIGURE 9.3
Four substances commonly consumed by those engaging in pica all demonstrate a dose-dependent capacity to absorb the antibiotic ciprofloxacin (10 ug/mL) in vitro. Redrawn from Ofoeule et al. 1999; reprinted by permission of *Annual Review of Nutrition.*

an antibiotic, ciprofloxacin (Ofoefule and Okonta 1999) (fig. 9.3). Indeed, all of these substances adsorbed significant quantities of the antibiotic.

ICE

It's easy to see how less-frequently reported pica substances fit with this hypothesis. Paper, for example, can contain both starch and clay. Baby powders contain starch and talc, a clay mineral. Plaster and chalk are also both dry and highly absorptive. There is one item that just doesn't belong, and that's ice.

At this point, it's not clear how, exactly, ice fits under this hypothesis, or if it does at all. One potential explanation is that ice is attractive because it is crunchy like many of the other craved items. Given that it binds so little, it may simply be a nonadaptive substitute that fits the bill because of its texture. A second explanation could be that ice does not itself prevent the entry of toxins or pathogens into the body, but rather, it treats one of the symptoms that result from their invasion: fever (Paul Sherman, personal communication). A third possibility relates to **glossitis**, the swelling of the tongue. Glossitis is a symptom of both inflammation and anemia (among other things), both of which are associated with pica. Ice can reduce the swelling of the tongue, so this may also explain the relationship.

To summarize data relevant to Prediction 9, a number of typical pica substances, including earth, charcoal, and starch, have the capacity to shield us from harmful effects of toxins and pathogens. Other pica substances like paper, plaster, and baby powder contain clay minerals and starches, and so thus may also be able to offer protection. Ice, however, does not seem to be able to perform such a function.

Prediction 10. Pica Would Occur More Frequently During Exposure to Toxins and Pathogens

If pica is a protective behavior, we would also expect non-food items to be eaten during periods of exposure to toxins and/or pathogens. These would include instances when toxic chemicals are ingested, when pathogens have been ingested, and/or in areas of the world that pathogens are particularly dense.

WHEN TOXIC FOODS ARE CONSUMED

Indeed, there are a number of examples of clays being consumed together with food containing poisonous levels of plant secondary compounds. Much of the work on this topic has been conducted by Drs. Johns and Duquette (Johns 1986; Johns 1996; Johns and Duquette 1991a, 1991b).

Take, for example, traditional methods of food preparation among the Pomo Indians in California and native Sardinians in Italy, which involve making bread out of acorn flour (Johns and Duquette 1991a, 1991b). Normally, acorns are dangerous to humans because they contain toxic levels of tannins. And tannins are heat stable, which means that even cooking cannot destroy them. So how can they be made safe? In both societies, the acorn meat is processed with clay, which binds the offending secondary compound, thereby making its consumption both safer and tastier. Wild potatoes are another type of food with which clays are eaten (Bourke et al.

1884; Laufer 1930; Stevenson 1908; Whiting 1939). Solanine, the glycoalkaloid most common in wild potatoes, is also heat stable. But clay can bind it, thereby preventing it from entering our bloodstream. This would explain why Indians of the American Southwest and Mexico have long consumed clays with wild potatoes, and some still do so in Peru and Bolivia today (Johns 1986; Johns 1996).

These and other examples led Johns to conclude that "geophagy is the most basic human detoxification technique" (Johns 1986:636). He goes on to discuss how the detoxification function provides an alternative explanation to the consumption of soil during famines: the soil was not consumed to fill the belly, but instead to counteract the toxins from the harmful leaves, plants, and roots that people had resorted to eating. In other words, the consumption of clay during famines may make items that are otherwise toxic, like bark and weeds, safe.

Humans aren't the only ones who use non-food substances to detoxify their food; Amazonian parrots (discussed above) and Zanzibar red colobus monkeys (fig. 9.4) do, too. Although Zanzibar red colobus monkeys are endangered and their absolute numbers are dwindling, they have been observed living in startlingly high population densities near some villages. Drs. Thomas Struhsaker and Kirstin Siex, biologists, and Dr. David Cooney, a toxicologist, have proposed that this density may be attributable in part to a habit seldom seen among other primates: the consumption of charcoal stolen from human settlements (Cooney and Struhsaker 1997; Struhsaker et al. 1997). Among these colobus monkeys, charcoal is highly sought after; juveniles wrestle one another for possession of a hunk of it, and older monkeys snatch it from younger ones.

Drs. Struhsaker and Cooney suggested that the consumption of charcoal helps monkeys to consume what would otherwise be toxic materials: the leaves of the Indian almond and mango trees. These leaves comprise a significant part of the colobus's diet, but they are high in phenolics, another potentially harmful plant secondary compound, which means that under normal circumstances they can only be eaten in limited quantities. It seems that thanks to their habit of eating charcoal, these clever little monkeys are able to exploit the leaves of two species that are high in protein and total phenolics better than they could in the absence of charcoal consumption.

While consumption of clays along with toxic substances provide tidy examples of detoxification, they are not examples of pica. The use of clay with acorn flour and wild potatoes is not a craving, it is part of a recipe. Furthermore, most pica does not occur in conjunction with the ingestion

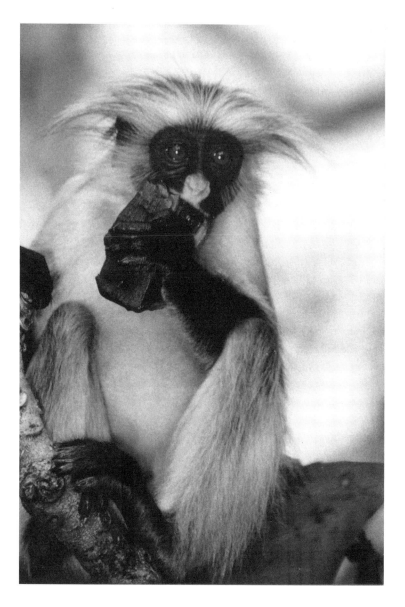

FIGURE 9.4
Juvenile Zanzibar red colobus monkey with piece of charcoal. Photo © generously provided by T. Struhsaker.

of toxic foods, or even any food in particular. When we surveyed Pembans about the circumstances under which they ate pica from among options including, upon awakening, *before food*, *with food*, *after food*, the overwhelming majority responded "just any time" (unpublished data). Ethnographic evidence corroborates this elsewhere. For example, the Ibo of Nigeria "swallow it at intervals during the day" (Basden 1938:171), and in the Antilles it is eaten "during all hours of the day" (Levacher 1840:255). Therefore, it is necessary to search further for an explanation of pica.

DURING GASTROINTESTINAL DISTRESS

You now know that nausea, vomiting, and diarrhea are a good indication of exposure to toxins and pathogens. It is therefore reasonable to expect that we would see non-food ingestion spike during periods of gastrointestinal distress. And indeed, it seems to.

Those simultaneously scary and adorable mountain gorillas in Rwanda provide an example of this. Diane Fossey described how the gorillas' "soil-eating binges in the dry months" created "vast caves" (1983:52). During the dry season, preferred food sources wither away, and they must resort to consuming more bamboo shoots than usual, which have high levels of cyanide-producing compounds that cause diarrhea. Dr. William Mahaney, a soil scientist, and colleagues at York University in Toronto, analyzed the soil that Rwandan gorillas ate (Mahaney et al. 1993). They determined that it was clay-rich, "similar to Kaopectate," and was therefore attributable to the treatment of diarrhea. This explanation is consistent with the detoxification hypothesis. Think back to the levels of analysis described in chapter 2. The reduction of diarrhea could be the trigger, or proximate cause, of geophagy, while the protection of intestinal integrity could be the ultimate one.

There are many anecdotes in which pica is associated with nausea (Brunhuber 2008; Swerdlow 2000; Walker et al. 1985). Although the least informative type of data, these anecdotes are nonetheless useful because they lend support to the plausibility of the detoxifying capacity of pica. Let us not forget that the consumption of earth in response to gastrointestinal distress is not pica, either; it's a phenomenon closer to self-medication.

When we look at patterns in "real" pica behavior, when non-food substances are craved, it's noteworthy that pica has been documented among two other populations who also regularly experience nausea and other forms of gastrointestinal distress: those with celiac disease (Kalayci et al. 2005) and renal dialysis patients (Ward and Kutner 1999). In one study, when celiac patients were put on gluten-free diets (which leads to a decrease in intestinal inflammation), their geophagy spontaneously ceased (Korman 1990). Further evidence of association between gastrointestinal distress and pica comes from Pemba, where amylophagy and geophagy occurred more frequently among pregnant women who experienced diarrhea or abdominal pain than it did among those without (Young et al. 2010a).

But what about pica that occurs when no obviously toxic items are consumed and in the absence of nausea and vomiting? This still needs explaining, which brings us to the next corollary, that pica would vary by region of the world.

IN TROPICAL CLIMATES

If pica is protective, we would anticipate finding it where people are exposed to increased levels of toxins or pathogens. Pathogens are not distributed equally around the world; foodborne pathogens multiply more rapidly in hot, humid, tropical climates than they do in temperate or cold ones (Hui et al. 2001a). Furthermore, species of pathogens and infectious diseases are most diverse nearest to the equator (Guernier et al. 2004). Thus, we would expect more pica to occur in humid tropical areas, i.e., at low altitudes near the equator.

We tested this hypothesis on geophagy using the Pica Literature Database.[6] First we categorized all reports of geophagy by climate type, using the **Köppen climate classification system.** We then classified what anthropologists consider to be a representative sample of world cultures, the **Standard Cross-Cultural Sample** (Murdock and White 1969), using this same climate classification system. In case the Standard Cross-Cultural Sample was not representative, we also plotted the distribution of the world population by climate type (Staszewski 1963). In order to reject this prediction about pica being more likely to occur in tropical climates, we would expect the distribution of world cultures across climate types to resemble the climactic distribution of geophagy.

Although geophagy occurs throughout the world, it is especially common in tropical climate zones and rare in polar and cold climates (fig. 9.5). In fact, the proportion of cultures in tropical areas that practice geophagy is much higher than would be predicted by either the distribution of cultural

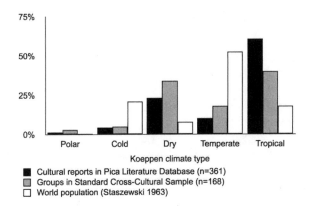

FIGURE 9.5
Distribution of geophagic cultures in Pica Literature Database, Standard Cross-Culture Sample, and world population distribution, by climate type. Geophagy occurs significantly more frequently in tropical climates than predicted by population distribution.

groups in the Standard Cross-Cultural Sample (p < 0.0001) or the worldwide population distribution by climate region (p < 0.0001). In short, for geophagy this corollary holds true; it cannot be rejected.

Prediction 11. Pica Would Occur More Frequently During Increased Susceptibility to the Harmful Effects of Toxins and Pathogens

Finally, under the protection-detoxification hypothesis, people would also engage in pica when they were most *susceptible* to the harmful effects of toxins and pathogens. Particularly susceptible life stages are those during which rapid cell division is occurring, i.e., periods of rapid growth: pregnancy and preadolescence (Bearer 1995). Furthermore, pregnant women are more susceptible to harm by toxins and pathogens because they are immuno-suppressed (Fessler 2002; Flaxman and Sherman 2000). Their immune system ramps down to avoid rejecting the embryo (remember the fetus is not only their genetic material; half of it is "foreign"—the father's). So avoidance of parasites and pathogens is especially important for the woman's own health during gestation. Therefore, this hypothesis predicts the occurrence of pica among pregnant women and children more commonly than any other age or sex groups.

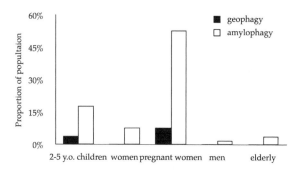

FIGURE 9.6
The prevalence of geophagy and amylophagy by life stage in Pemba; it is significantly higher among pregnant women.

There is plenty of anecdotal evidence that pica is strongly associated with pregnancy (chapters 1, 4, 7). Remarks made during ethnographic interviews in Pemba reinforced this. When I asked one woman what caused her to eat uncooked rice and earth, she pointed accusatorily at her baby and said, "He caused it! It left me as soon as he did!" More robust evidence backs this up, too. When we look at the geophagy scores from the Pica Literature Database, we see that this hypothesis correctly predicts the highest geophagy score among pregnant women (fig. 2.2, p. 30). Furthermore, the group with the second-highest geophagy score, preadolescents, also fits this prediction. In Pemba, the distribution of geophagy and amylophagy indicates similar peaks in pregnancy and childhood (fig. 9.6).

The protection-detoxification hypothesis further predicts that pica would be more likely to occur early in pregnancy, during embryogenesis (Flaxman and Sherman 2000), when tissues are most susceptible to damage from teratogens (Moore and Persaud 1998). There are some anecdotes that suggest that pica is found primarily in early pregnancy, such as this little gem from 1663: "Women with child use to be freed of this disease [pica] about the fourth month, because then the Child is grown greater, and so consumeth more of the humors, and the mother has sent forth by often vomitings; but if it last longer, 'tis dangerous" (Riverius et al. 1663).

In the Pica Literature Database, we were able to identify only fifteen reports in which the timing of pica within pregnancy was explicit. In those, the majority of the accounts that discussed the timing of geophagy during pregnancy indicated that consumption occurred during the first trimester (cf. fig. 8.2, p. 103). This is a small number of reports, so caution should be used when making conclusions based on this data.[7] In general, however, the demographic patterns in pica are correctly predicted by this hypothesis.

In this chapter, we have seen that many pica substances are good at shielding us from the harmful effects of chemicals and pathogens. As predicted, non-food substances are consumed in conjunction with the consumption of toxic chemicals and during gastrointestinal distress. Stronger evidence of the protective capacity of earth is the increased prevalence of it in tropical climates, where pathogen densities are higher. And finally, we have seen that those who can handle toxins or pathogens least well, pregnant women and preadolescents, engage in pica the most frequently. Paradoxically, "dirt," it seems, may have a cleansing effect.

CHAPTER TEN

Putting the Pica Pieces Together

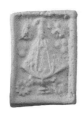 IN THIS book, it has been my intention to answer Mama Khadija's question (cf. preface) by way of guiding you through the centuries of history, range of opinion, and myriad of available data about pica. As we have seen, it is a rich and multifaceted behavior; it spans the centuries and the continents, influencing, and being influenced by, both cultural expectations and biological constraints and opportunities. In this final chapter, I'd like to take a step back and look at what we know from a more global perspective. This, in turn, makes it possible to identify gaps in our knowledge. Taking stock of what we don't know is useful for selecting the most fruitful directions in future work on non-food cravings.

What We Know

Pica is ubiquitous. There is evidence that pica is hundreds of thousands, if not millions, of years old (chapter 1). It happens in almost every country and is found with greatest frequency among pregnant women and young children (chapters 1, 6, and 9).

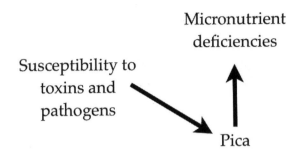

FIGURE 10.1
A potential relationship between pica, micronutrient deficiencies, and protection.

Pica may be adaptive. Pica has been dismissed as pathological and aberrant for many centuries (chapters 5 and 6). However, there is good reason to believe that it is somehow adaptive. It is found throughout the animal kingdom (chapters 1 and 9) and a number of pica substances have healing or medicinal properties (chapters 3, 4, and 9).

Pica is not due to hunger. It is clear that very little pica is explained by a shortage of food (chapter 7). Few people are consuming earth, starch, or ice out of hunger.

Pica is unlikely to contribute micronutrients to the diet. In terms of micronutrient supplementation, although the currently available data are limited in quality and quantity, they suggest that the elimination of a micronutrient deficiency does not cause the cessation of pica and that most pica substances are an unlikely source of micronutrients (chapter 8).

Pica may cause micronutrient deficiencies. At present, it seems plausible that the association between most forms of pica and micronutrient deficiencies is caused by pica substances themselves. They prevent micronutrient absorption, either by binding to ingested food or coating the intestine, making absorption more difficult (chapter 8; see also fig. 10.1).

Pica may protect and detoxify. At this point, the best supported explanation of the adaptive function of pica is that it functions to protect and detoxify (chapter 9; also fig. 10.1). Experimental data indicate that at least some pica substances are capable of shielding us from damage that would otherwise be inflicted by harmful chemicals and pathogens. Furthermore, the demographic profile of those who engage in pica most frequently, pregnant women and young children living in the tropics, is also consistent with this hypothesis.

What We Don't Know

While there are now thousands of documents about pica, there is still much unknown. In order to structure our (lack of) knowledge, I return to Tinbergen's Four Questions (cf. chapter 2).

Causation

The mechanistic causes of pica have not received much attention. What are the specific changes that occur during iron or zinc deficiency that could trigger pica? Do smell or taste sensitivities to compounds in pica substances change as iron or zinc levels fluctuate? We know that some women attribute the cause of their pica to pregnancy, but what is it about pregnancy that triggers pica? Do hormonal fluctuations alter taste or smell sensitivity? And if so, what compounds do pregnant women become more sensitive to? Many have commented on the appeal of petrichor, the smell of damp earth—what is it that they smell? Might it be the compound geosmin? Could changes in the functioning of the digestive tract drive pica? Pica also occurs outside of pregnancy; is the mechanism then different than during pregnancy? Identifying a physiological mechanism by which pica occurs would greatly strengthen current explanations.

Development

This type of question deals with how behavior changes with age. We have cross-sectional data on subsets of a population (e.g., schoolchildren, pregnant women), but we have very little on the distribution of pica within an entire community. In other words, we know, for example, if children in a community eat earth, but not if the adult males or non-pregnant women there do; very few studies have measured pica across more than one sex or age group. It would also be useful to track pica longitudinally (i.e., throughout people's lives) to see when these behaviors wax and wane within an individual. Not only would such data provide more accurate information than behaviors recalled from childhood, it could be linked to our understanding of developmental biology to yield new insights into functions of pica.

Evolutionary Origins

Although there are many reports of non-food consumption by other species (chapter 1), they are irregular in quality and content. For example, we know very little about the conditions under which birds, reptiles, and mammals engage in pica. Are they pregnant? Sick? Have they ingested toxins? Is it a seasonal behavior? This type of information coupled with data about their digestive tract and metabolic requirements would be extremely useful for distinguishing differences and commonalities in the function(s) of pica across species. We also know little about the selection process of soils that animals deem fit for consumption, nor if they would be willing to ingest other pica substances, such as charcoal or starch, when suitable earth is not available.

Functional Consequences

We have more information on functional consequences of pica than we do on the others types of questions, but even so, it is scant. At this point, for pica, available data only permit the study of its observed effects on illness frequency and to speculate about the plausibility of its effects on other conditions. We have some idea about short-term consequences of pica on micronutrient status, but we know very little about the effect of pica substances on other aspects of health. For example, it would be extremely useful to measure the timing and effect of pica substances with respect to subclinical indices of inflammation, i.e., indicators that measure health problems that a person might not be aware of, such as acute phase proteins. We also know almost nothing about the effect of pica on the prevention of adverse gestational outcomes, e.g., miscarriage. Future research into the functional consequences of pica has real potential to improve our capacity to respond to chemical and pathogenic challenges through a better understanding of the protective and detoxification functions of clay, starch, and charcoal.

Why We Need to Know It

Some of these questions about pica are new and reflect our modern understanding of biology and culture, while many of them are old, even ancient. No matter their age, it is clear they are complex and challenging. And now, more than ever, it is important for us to answer them.

If there is one message you take away from this book, it is that pica is very much alive, affecting the lives of hundreds of thousands of people each and every day, many of them in the most vulnerable segments of our societies. This would not be a problem if we knew for certain that they were protecting themselves from harmful chemicals and pathogens. In fact, if we could unequivocally prove this hypothesis, we might be able to recommend pica as a cost-effective preventative medicine that actually improves people's lives. Unfortunately, there is the very real possibility that pica decreases the availability of essential micronutrients and is a harmful practice that should be stopped. In either scenario, knowing the definitive consequences of pica has the potential to affect the lives of many.

But there is another reason to continue the quest to understand pica, and that is that it is a phenomenon at the heart of the complex biocultural being that is us humans. Pica has deep roots both in the microscopic world of cells and tissues that make up our bodies as well as in the complex workings of the macroscopic world, the culture that is the foundation of our societies. In essence, studying pica is a way to study what it means to be *us*.

It has been my desire and privilege to stand on the proverbial shoulders of the hundreds of scholars of pica to spark your interest in this fascinating enigma. In his 1930 monograph on geophagy, Berthold Laufer wrote that "if these pages should have the good fortune to attract the attention . . . to stimulate a fresh investigation of the problems involved, I should feel amply rewarded for the trouble and time I have taken in gathering this material" (Laufer 1930:108). Eighty years later, I couldn't agree more.

Notable Moments
in the History of Pica

YEAR	EVENT
2 million years ago	Archeological evidence of geophagy by *Homo habilis* (Clark 2001:659–62).
~400 B.C.E.	Hippocrates provides first written account of pica: "If a pregnant woman wants to eat earth or charcoal, and eats it, the infant will show signs of those things on its head" (Hippocrates 1853:487).
~300 B.C.E.	The Greek philosopher Aristotle speculates on causes of non-food cravings: "Other such states again are the results of a morbid disposition or of habit, as, e.g., the practice of plucking out one's hair, or biting one's nails, or eating cinders and earth, or of committing unnatural vices" (Aristotle 1897: Bk. 7, p. 220).
30 C.E.	Cornelius Celsus, a Roman physician, documents the first association between anemia and pica: "They who, without jaundice, have a bad complexion for some considerable time, are plagued with pains of the head, or have a morbid appetite for earth" (Celsus 1831:39).
70 C.E.	Scholars Pliny the Elder and Dioscorides provide the first written accounts of medicinal properties of terra sigillata (Dioscorides et al. 1934: Bk. 5, ch. 113; Pliny/ Rackham 1952: Bk. 18, ch. 29).
2nd century	The Greek physician Soranus uses the term "kissa" (meaning jaybird) to describe non-food cravings in pregnant women (Soranus 1956: Bk. 1, ch. 15, p. 49; Weiss-Amer 1993).
167 C.E.	Galen witness the extraction of terra sigillatta on Lemnos (in Brock 1929:194).
4th century	The Greek physician Oribasius suggests that dry starch is especially beneficial for women who crave earth or are nauseated (Oribasius et al. 1851: Bk. 5, ch. 1).

6th century	Aetius of Amida provides the first written use of the term "pica." He also expands the list of non-foods craved by pregnant women, to include egg shells and ashes (Aetius of Amida/Ricci 1542 [1950]: Bk. 16, ch. 10, pp. 20–21).
980	The Persian physician Avicenna recommended treating pica with "iron steeped in fine wine and strained through a Hippocratic sleeve" (in Cooper 1957:10).
11th century	Trotula of Salerno described geophagy as a common but treatable problem for pregnant women: "If, however, she desires clay or chalk or coals, let beans cooked with sugar be given to her" (Green 2001:97).
13th century	Marco Polo described Christians using red earth from St. Thomas Aquinas's tomb in India as a remedy for a variety of illnesses (Marco Polo et al. 1863:267).
1581	Accused thief Wendel Thumblardt demonstrates on himself the power of terra sigillata to prevent death from mercury poisoning and was freed from jail (in Thompson 1914:436).
1606	First of 25 *dissertatios* on pica written by medical students throughout western Europe is published (Muccius and Hartmannus 1606).
1617	Famine in Germany caused people to eat earth; the hill that was source of the earth collapsed, killing 5 (Strose and Suhle 1891:7).
1663	The first written observation of pagophagy was made by French physician Lazarus Riverius: women and young girls suffering from chlorosis eating large quantities of ice and snow (Riverius et al. 1663: Bk. 9, pp. 248–79; Bk. 15, pp. 400–405).
1816	Penitente Bernardo Abeyta builds the Santuario de Chimayo in New Mexico
1870	Livingstone describes anemia in Zanzibar as "the disease of earth-eating" (Livingstone and Waller 1875:346).
1930	Laufer publishes the first anthropological monograph on geophagy (Laufer 1930).
1968	First experiments on the ability of clays (Minnich et al. 1968) and starches (Blum et al. 1968) to inhibit micronutrient absorption.
2004	First double-blind randomized control study of the effect of micronutrient supplementation on geophagy is published (Nchito et al. 2004).

Prevalence of Pica Among Representative Populations of Pregnant Women (n=47)[a]

Population	Location	N	Prevalence of pica[b]	Reference
Women attending antenatal clinics	Pemba Island, Tanzania	2,361	Any: 40.1%; starch, 36.3%; earth, 5.2%	Young et al. 2010
Pregnant and lactating women attending two health facilities	Dar es Salaam, Tanzania	204	Any pica: 63.7%; earth, 60.0%; ice, 16.1%; ash, 15.4%; other, <3%	Nyaruhucha 2009
HIV+ pregnant women enrolled in Vitamin A trial	Dar es Salaam, Tanzania	971	Earth: 29%	Antelman et al. 2000; Kawai et al. 2009
Recent parturients	Buenos Aires, Argentina	327	Any pica: 21.9%	Lopez et al. 2001; Lopez et al. 2007
Nationally representative sample of pregnant women	Denmark	70,000	Any pica (earth, chalk, paper, other): 0.02%	Mikkelsen et al. 2006
Women in second trimester participating in longitudinal intervention cohort study	Nyanza province, western Kenya	827	Earth: 45.7% during pregnancy; 30.6% at 3 m postpartum; 25.5% at 6 m postpartum	Luoba et al. 2005
Ganda ethnic group who had delivered at government hospital	Kampala, Uganda	59	Earth: 51%	Wakou 2003
Recent parturients in hospital obstetric unit	Zaria, Nigeria	200	Earth: 50%	Sule and Madugu 2001

Women attending rural antenatal health clinics	North Carolina, USA	128	Any pica: 38%; ice, 36.7%; starch, 4.7%; earth, 1.6%	Corbett et al. 2003
Healthy women attending antenatal clinics, 16 w gestational age	Shiraz, Iran	270	Earth: 28.3%	Karimi et al. 2002
Gravidae or recent parturients at outpatient clinics	Southern California & Ensenada, Mexico	225	Any pica (earth, ice, ash, other): 33.1%	Simpson et al. 2000
Women attending 4 antenatal clinics	Accra, Ghana	502	Earth: 28.5%; starch, 3.6%; chalk, 1.2%	Tayie and Lartey 1999
Participants in WIC[a] program	Houston and Prairie View, Tex., USA	281	Any pica: 76.5%; ice/frost, 68.3%; other, 8.2%	Rainville 1998
Women attending antenatal clinics	Kilfi District Hospital, Coastal Kenya	275	Earth: 56%	Geissler et al. 1998b
Women attending antenatal clinics	Katima Mulilo clinic, Eastern Caprivi, Namibia	171	Earth: 44.4%	Thomson 1997
Randomly selected pregnant women from 3 health centers	Riyadh, Saudi Arabia	321	Any pica (clay, ice, paper, other): 8.8%	Al-kanhal and Bani 1995
Women delivering at hospital	Midwestern USA	300	Any pica: 64.7%	Cooksey 1995
Rural antenatal clinic attendees at health department	Muscogee County, Ga., USA	125	Any pica: 14.4%; ice, 6.4%; earth, 4%; starch, 4%; other, 6.4%	Smulian et al. 1995
Pregnant women 13–24 y	Camden, N.J., USA	1,334	Ice: 53%; other (predominantly starch), 7%	Coles et al. 1995
Pregnant women 16–35 y at antenatal clinics and hospitals	Washington, D.C., USA	553	Any pica (ice, frost, starch, other): 8.1%	Edwards et al. 1994
Pregnant women attending antenatal clinics	Nakuru district, Kenya	422	Earth or charcoal: 45.0%	Mbati-Mwaka 1993

Recent parturients	Atlanta, Ga., USA	109	Ice: 18.3%; earth, 2.7%; starch, 2.7%; other, 1%	Kirsch 1990
Antenatal and postpartum clinics at university hospitals	Kinshasa, Zaire	802	Earth: 71.3%	Tandu-Umba and Paluku 1988
Pregnant women at 2 antenatal clinics	Mobile, Ala., USA	120	Any pica: 20%; starch, 16.7%; clay, 4.2%	Sharp-Ross 1987
Pregnant and recently delivered women	Greater Khartoum, Sudan	416	Any pica: 13.6%	Osman 1985
Community recruitment of women from 5 racial groups with infants <1 y	South Africa	1771	Any pica (earth, ash, ice, chalk, other): 24.0%	Walker et al. 1985
County-sponsored antenatal clinics	Maryland, USA	60	Any pica (ice, burnt matches): 11.7%	Schwab and Axelson 1984
Private and public antenatal clinics	Kingston, Jamaica	125	Ice: 11.2%; earth, 4.8%; ash, 2.4%; other, 5.6%	Landman and Hall 1989; Landman and Hall 1992
Women in community, retrospective about behavior during pregnancy	El Campo, Tex., USA	155	Starch or earth: 33%	Taylor 1979
Random sample of pregnant women receiving care	University of Virginia Medical Center, Charlottesville. Va., USA	85	Baking soda: 8%	Thomas 1978
WIC[a] clients	Pitt County, N.C., USA	53	Any pica: 17.0%	Mansfield 1977
Patients at public clinic	Ingham County, Mich., USA	40	Any pica (starch, clay, other): 30.0%	Snowdon 1977
Women admitted for delivery	Mysore, India	500	Any pica (earth, ash, charcoal, raw rice): 18%	Khanum 1976
Women in active labor at Cook County Hospital	Chicago, Ill., USA	623	Starch: 24.4%	Keith et al. 1975
Pregnant women	St. Louis, Mo., USA	100	Any pica: 43%	Wilks 1974

Consecutive patients at antenatal clinics	Georgia, USA	410	Any pica (starch, chalk, clay): 16%	Bronstein and Dollar 1974
Primigravidae	Norway	84	Any pica: 33%	Jameson 1971
Women in active labor at Cook County Hospital	Chicago, Ill., USA	987	Starch: 34.6%	Keith et al. 1968
Randomly selected postnatal inpatients	Urban and rural areas of Augusta, Ga., USA	200	Any pica: 55%; earth, 32.5%; starch, 19%; other, 3.5%	O'Rourke et al. 1967
Consecutive pregnant women	Philadelphia, Pa., USA	50	Starch: 26%	Sage 1962
Obstetric patients in 5 y longitudinal study	Nashville, Tenn., USA	571	Starch: 17%; other, <1%	Payton et al. 1960
Recent parturients	City County Hospital Dallas, Tex., USA	100	Earth: 18%; starch, 7%; baking powder, 4%	Gladfelter et al. 1960
Letters from BBC listeners after a broadcast about pica during pregnancy	Great Britain, mostly England	—	In 509 letters, 187 cravings for non-food substances were described	Harries and Hughes 1958
Consecutive women in third trimester, lower income	Harlem, N.Y., USA	600	Starch: 19.2%; ice, 5.2%; clay, 1.5%	Posner et al. 1957
Women attending antenatal clinics	Georgia and Alabama, USA	211	Earth, starch, or paper: 21.0% during pregnancy, 10.4% when not pregnant	Edwards et al. 1954
Lower-income women seeking antenatal care at county clinics	11 counties in southern Mississippi, USA	361	Earth: 38.5%; starch, 25.2%	Ferguson and Keaton 1950

[a] *Abbreviations:* d—day(s), m—month(s), y—year(s), WIC—The Special Supplemental Program for Women, Infants, and Children

[b] Substances most frequently consumed are listed if described by study. When >3 items are consumed by participants, "other" is used. "Any pica" without a description following indicates that pica substances were not specified.

Prevalence of Pica Among Representative Populations of Children (n=11)[a]

Population	Location	N	Prevalence of pica[b]	Reference
Schoolchildren 7–15 y	Lusaka, Zambia	406	Earth 74.4%	Nchito et al. 2004
Schoolchildren 8–14 y	KwaZulu Natal, South Africa	1,161	Earth: 47%	Saathoff et al. 2002
Representative sample of children <5 y	3 villages in Khombole, Senegal	275	Earth: 58.7%	Diouf et al. 2000
Representative random sample of children 1–10 y	Two upstate N.Y. counties, USA	659	Any pica: 1.7%	Marchi and Cohen 1990
Random sample of children 10–18 y	Western Kenya	156	Earth: 73.1%	Geissler et al. 1998a
Children 13–60 m	Sirjon county, Iran	212	Any pica: 15.6%	Rokni 1990
Children 8 m to 7 y	Richmond, Va., USA	2,402	Plaster or paint chips: 9.0%	De la Burde and Reames 1973
Interviews with parents of randomly selected children & mailed surveys	Boston, Mass., USA	186; 1,000	Any pica (paper, earth, cloth, other): 18.5% in last 14 d	Barltrop 1966
Children 1–6 y at a private and a public clinic	Washington, D.C., USA	780	Any pica: 23.8%	Millican et al. 1962
Children living in low-income area	Baltimore, Md., USA	333	Any pica: 69.6%	Bradley and Bessman 1958
Schoolchildren	Mississippi, USA	207	Earth: 26%	Dickins and Ford 1942

[a] *Abbreviations:* d—day(s), m—month(s), y—year(s)
[b] Substances most frequently consumed are listed if described by study. When >3 items are consumed by participants, "other" is appended. "Any pica" without a description following indicates that pica substances were not specified.

Pica in Literature

Source (alphabetical by author)	Passage Description	Quotes
Before Night Falls (Arenas 2000 [1992])	A memoir by a Cuban dissident and author, in which he recalls eating earth in early life.	I was two. I was standing there, naked. I bent down and licked the earth. The first taste I remember is the taste of the earth. I used to eat dirt with my cousin Dulce Maria, who was also two. I was a skinny kid with a distended belly full of worms from eating so much dirt. We ate dirt in the shed. (p. 1)

I should make it clear right away that to eat dirt is not a metaphor, or a sensational act. All the country kids did it. It has nothing to do with magic realism, or anything of the sort. One had to eat something, dirt was the only thing we had plenty of, and perhaps that was why we ate it. (p. 11)

One of the first things I ever did in my life was to eat dirt. (p. 27) |
| *World's End* (Boyle 1987) | Depeyster Van Wart is a wealthy businessman with distinguished ancestors who eats earth when he is nervous. Van Wart helps himself to pinches of his ancestral earth, taken neat or sprinkled on sandwiches and in tea, on pages 33, 36–39, 68, 123, 152, 158, 284, and 480, | Depeyster Van Wart, twelfth heir to Van Wart Manor, the late seventeenth-century country house that lay just outside Peterskill on Van Wart Ridge where it commanded a sweeping view of the town dump and the rushing, refuse-clogged waters of Van Wart Creek, was a terraphage. That is, he ate dirt. Nothing so common as leaf mold or carpet dust, but a very particular species of dirt, bone-dry and smelling faintly of the deaths of the trillions of microscopic creatures that gave it body and substance, dirt that hadn't seen the light of day in three hundred years |

	usually in times of stress, such as dealing with his obnoxious daughter or negotiating land acquisitions.	and silted cool and sterile through the fingers, as rarefied in its way as the stuff trapped beneath the temple at Angkor Wat or moldering in Grant's Tomb. No, what he ate was ancestral dirt, scooped with a garden digger from the cool weatherless caverns beneath the house. Even now, as he sat idly at his ceremonial desk behind the frosted glass door at Depeyster Manufacturing, thinking of lunch, the afternoon paper and the acquisition of property, the business envelope in his breast pocket was half-filled with it. From time to time, ruminative, he would wet the tip of his forefinger and dip it furtively into the envelope before bringing it to his lips. (p. 33)
The Good Earth (Buck 1994 [1931])	Wang Lung, the protagonist, and his family are slowly starving to death.	The extreme gnawing in his stomach which he had had in his stomach at first was past and he could stir up a little of the earth from a certain spot in one of his fields and give it to the children without desiring any of it for himself. This earth they had been eating in water for some days—goddess of mercy earth, it was called, because it had some slight nutritious quality in it, although in the end it could not sustain life. But made into a gruel it allayed the children's hunger for some time and put something into their distended, empty bellies. (p. 84)
Don Quixote (pt. 1, 1605; pt. 2, 1615) (Cervantes et al. 2003)	Anselmo becomes so strongly obsessed with testing the chastity of his love, Camila, that he compares the strength of his obsession to the longing that some anemic women have for non-food substances. He insists that his best friend, Lotario, try to seduce Camila to ascertain her faithfulness. Things end terribly: Camila	Assuming this, you must consider that I suffer now from the disease that afflicts some women, filling them with the desire to eat earth, plaster, charcoal and other things that are even worse, and sickening to look at, let alone to eat; therefore it is necessary to use some artifice to cure me, and this could be done with ease if you simply start, even if indifferently and falsely, to woo Camila. (pp. 411–12)

	and Lotario fall in love and Anselmo dies of a broken heart. After Lotario dies in battle, Camila enters a convent.	
Salad Fingers (Firth 2004)	Salad Fingers is the main character of this dark, Flash cartoon series. He is a bald, hunchbacked humanoid with light-green skin, and no visible nose or ears and long, strangely shaped fingers. He appears to suffer from psychosis, and is unable or unwilling to distinguish between living beings and inanimate objects. He often assigns such objects proper names and appears to believe that they can communicate with him directly, sometimes voicing their perceived thoughts himself. He lives alone in a small shack with the number 22 on the door. One of his habits is tasting dirt, which he calls "floor-sugar" (Wikipedia 2009).	
One Hundred Years of Solitude (García Márquez 1998 [1967])	Rebeca arrives at the house of the Buendía family as a traumatized 11-year-old orphan, with her parents bones clattering in a bag.	No one understood why she had not died of hunger until the Indians, who were aware of everything, for they went ceaselessly about the house on their stealthy feet, discovered that Rebecca only liked to eat the damp earth of the courtyard and the cake of whitewash that she picked off the walls with her nails. (p. 46)

Later, as a teenager, she falls madly in love with the pianola instructor, Pietro Crespi. When he leaves Macondo, she is utterly lovesick:

She would put handfuls of earth in her pockets, and ate them in small bits without being seen, with a confused feeling of pleasure and rage, as she instructed her girl friends in the most difficult needlepoint and spoke about other men, who did not deserve the sacrifice of having one eat the whitewash on the walls because of them. The handfuls of earth made the only man who deserved that show of degradation less remote and more certain, as if the ground that he walked on with his fine patent leather boots in another part of the world were transmitting to her the weight and the temperature of his blood in a mineral savor that left a harsh aftertaste in her mouth and a sediment of peace in her heart. (p. 69)

She is filled with anxiety as she waited for Pietro Crespi's letters which would arrive with the mail that came every two weeks. Once, when the mule did not come, she ate a very large quantity.

Mad with desperation, Rebeca got up in the middle of the night and ate handfuls of earth in the garden with a suicidal drive, weeping with pain and fury, chewing tender earthworms and chipping her teeth on snail shells. (p. 72)

After a tragedy puts her marriage to Pietro Crespi on indefinite pause, José Arcadio returns from adventures in the world and she is enveloped in a cloud of lust for him.

On a certain occasion José Arcadio looked at her body with shameless attention and said to her: "You're a woman, little sister." Rebeca lost control of herself. She went back to eating earth and the whitewash on the walls with the avidity of previous days, and she sucked her finger with so much anxiety that she developed a callus on her thumb. (p. 97)

Ellen Foster
(Gibbons 1988)

Ellen Foster, a young white girl whose mother has died and whose father is worse than useless, has a black friend, Starletta, who eats dirt.

Starletta and her mama both eat dirt. My daddy slapped my face for eating dirt. Oh yes but I have seen Starletta sucking in her face drawing what she can from red clay. My daddy slapped my face and jerked my elbow round to my nose and he ran his finger across my gums feeling for grit. She eats that mess like it is good to her. She sits at the end of the row while her mama chops. She loosens a piece and pops it in her jaw and

		squeezes. She sits and eats clay dirt and picks at her bug bites. Starletta has orange teeth and she will plait my hair if I ask her right. (p. 20)
Among the Pines or, South in secession-time (Gilmore 1862)	A black servant and his white master are discussing the living conditions of poor whites in rural Georgia with whom they had spent the night after getting caught in a flash flood.	"Mighty pore, massa. Niggas lib better'n dat." "Yes," I replied, "but these folks despise you blacks; they seem to be both poor and proud." "Yas, massa, dey'm pore 'cause dey wont work, and dey'm proud 'cause dey'r white. Dey wont work 'cause dey see de darky slaves doin' it, and tink it am beneaf white folks to do as de darkies do. Dis habin' slaves keeps dis hull country pore." "Who told you that?" I asked, astonished at hearing a remark showing so much reflection from a negro. "Nobody, massa; I see it myseff." "Are there many of these poor whites around Georgetown?" "Not many 'round Georgetown, sar, but great many in de up-country har, and dey'm all 'like—pore and no account; none ob 'em kin read, and dey all eat clay." "Eat clay!" I said; "what do you mean by that?" "Didn't you see, massa, how yaller all dem wimmin war? Dat's 'cause dey eat clay. De little children begin 'fore dey kin walk, and dey eat it till dey die; dey chaw it like 'backer. It makes all dar stumacs big, like as you seed 'em, and spiles dar 'gestion. It 'm mighty onhealfy." "Can it be possible that human beings do such things! The brutes wouldn't do that." "No, massa, but dey do it; dey'm pore trash. Dat's what de big folks call 'em, and it am true; dey'm long way lower down dan de darkies." (p. 82)
A Respectable Trade (Gregory 2007)	A slave who has named herself Died of Shame eats earth in order to kill herself after being brutally raped by Sir	"She will not eat food . . . She is eating . . ." "Earth?" he guessed. Frances's glance flew to his face. "You knew?"

Charles, a white trader. In a terrible irony, her owners, two English women, Frances and Miss Cole, then call on Sir Charles for a solution to her earth-eating.

He shrugged. "It's not unusual. A foul habit, isn't it? The women do it often. It makes them sick as dogs. They get the yaws, and they will eat it till they die sometimes. It is their mad spite. They know they are robbing you of their purchase price. They are insane with spite. You will need to use a bridle, ma'am."

"A bridle?"

He tutted in irritation. "Of course, you will not have one to hand. I had thought myself at home! We put a bridle on them when they eat soil. A metal cage which goes around the face, under the jaw, with a gag of metal across the mouth. Their driver must take it off at mealtimes and watch her to make sure she eats her food. She must wear it all the rest of the time. They are cunning as monkeys. If they want to eat dirt, they will get their hands on it somehow. The only way is to gag their mouths." "And you frequently use these devices?" Miss Cole asked, interested.

"We could not run the plantations without them." (pp. 154–56)

Frances later discovers the corpse of Shame.

Frances went forward and recoiled. She had forgotten the bridle. The young woman's face was encased in metal. Blood and saliva stained her neck from where the gag had cut her mouth and gums. She looked like a victim of some barbaric medieval torture. And Frances had ordered this. And now the woman was dead. (pp. 178–79)

The Raghuvamsha of Kalidasa (Kale 1997)

An epic 13th-century Indian poem that describes the greatness and ancestry of a long line of warrior kings. Queen Sudakshina, the mother of one such warrior king, eats clay during her pregnancy.

The king smelling, in private, her mouth fragrant with clay (that she would eat), never felt satisfaction, like an elephant smelling a pond in a forest tract, sprinkled over with drops from the clouds, at the close of summer.

Her future son was to enjoy the sovereignty of the earth with his conquering chariot stopping only at the extremities of the quarters, as the lord of the gods enjoys that of heaven; hence it was that she set her heart upon clay in preference to all other objects of taste.

154

"Through bashfulness the princess of
Magadha does not tell me her wish—what
are the things that she has a craving for?—"
thus did the lord of the North-Kosalas
constantly ask his wife's companions in
loving concern. (Canto III, nos. 3–5)

The Poisonwood Bible (Kingsolver 1998)	Orleanna, the mother of four daughters, is describing the emotional and financial hardships she encounters during pregnancy.	When I was carrying the twins I had such desperate cravings I sometimes went out at night on my hands and knees and secretly ate dirt from the garden. (p. 226)
	In the Congo, mourning mothers would eat dirt from the graves of their children.	The Reverend forbade us to observe any ritual over which he was not asked to preside, but twice, at night, I slipped out to spy on the funerals. Inside a grove of trees the mothers threw themselves on mounds of dirt that covered their children. Crawled on hands and knees, tried to eat the dirt from the graves. Other women had to pull the away. (p. 336)
"One View of the Question" (Kipling 1893)	This short story takes the form of a rather bigoted letter written by a fictional Muslim agent of a Shah, describing, among other things, his despisal of educated Bengalis.	Once more, there is a green-sickness upon all the people of this country. They eat dirt even now to stay their cravings. (p. 102; "green-sickness" is a synonym for *chlorosis*: *see* glossary)
Georgia scenes, characters, incidents, &c., in the first half century of the republic (Longstreet 1835)	Description of a character in a humorous sketch.	Now there happened to reside in the county just alluded to a fellow by the name of Ransy Sniffle: a sprout of Richmond, who, in his earlier days, had fed copiously upon red clay and blackberries. This diet had given to Ransy a complexion that a corpse would have disdained to own, and an abdominal rotundity that was quite unprepossessing. Long spells of the fever and ague, too, in Ransy's youth, had conspired with clay and blackberries to throw him quite out of the order of nature. His shoulders were fleshless and elevated; his head large and flat; his neck slim and translucent; and his arms, hands, fingers, and feet were lengthened out of all

proportion to the rest of his frame. His joints were large and his limbs small; and as for flesh, he could not, with propriety, be said to have any. (p. 43)

María, the Potter of San Ildefonso (Marriott 1948)

María Martinez (1887?–1980) was a potter who made the black-on-black San Ildefonso pottery famous. As a child, when she fell very sick, her mother made a promise that if she survived, they would walk to Chimayo. This pilgrimage, at age 10, is described in María's biography:

A groundskeeper took a bunch of keys that hung from his belt, selected one of them, and unlocked the door. Slowly one leaf of the door swung inward, and they went inside. . . . The child smelled an earthen dampness, like the darkness of the storeroom at home, and it surprised her. Most churches smelled of dry dust, not wet.

"There are steps going down," said Mother. "You must go down them. When you get to the bottom, take off all your clothes. Don't be afraid, because nobody can see you. Then take this holy medal and scrape off the earth on the sides of the hole. Rub the earth all over your body. That's what makes you well."

"Will you go with me?" María asked.

"Just you can go. This is your pilgrimage. After you have rubbed yourself with the sacred earth and dressed again, take the medal and dig out enough earth to fill your water bottle. That much you can take home with you, to drink there to make you well. While you are doing this, you should say your 'Our Father.' Don't think about any thing but your prayers and the Santo Nino." (p. 36)

In the Bengali play "Tazzab Byapar" (Mitra 1904)

A street vendor hawking baked clay cups and figures boasts how her cups of baked clay are "well burnt, very crisp to eat and, at the same time, cheap and that delicate ladies, who are about to become mothers, should at once buy them, as by eating the same they will be blessed with sons."

Paradise (Morrison 1998)	In a letter to her mother, Pat asks about a long car ride her mother and father took with some other couples.	Did Soane or Dovey, new brides too, talk woman talk with you? You thought you were pregnant again and so did they. So did you talk together about how you all felt? Make tea for hemorrhoids, give one another salt to lick or copper dirt to eat in secret? I craved baking soda when I carried Billie Delia. Did you when you carried me? (p. 200)
	Lone, an 86-year-old midwife, is bemoaning the fact that women in her town prefer to deliver in a hospital rather than at home with her assistance.	No matter she taught them how to comb their breasts to set the milk flowing; what to do with the afterbirth, what direction the knife under the mattress should point. No matter she searched the county to get them the kind of dirt they wanted to eat. No matter she had gotten in the bed with them, pressing the soles of her feet to theirs, helping them push, push! Or massaged their stomachs with sweet oil for hours. (p. 271)
Song of Solomon (Morrison 1987)	Ruth, impregnated by her husband with a baby he tried multiple times to abort, goes to seek consolation from a woman who knows a lot about birth, despite not having the scar of birth, a belly button, herself.	Pilate listened to Ruth's plight and sent her daughter to the store for a box of Argo cornstarch. She sprinkled a little of it into her hand and offered it to Ruth, who obediently took a lump and put it in her mouth. As soon as she tasted it, felt its crunchiness, she asked for more, and ate half a box before she left. (From then on she ate cornstarch, cracked ice, nuts, and once in a fit she put a few tiny pebbles of gravel in her mouth. "When you expectin, you have to eat what the baby craves," Pilate said, "less it come in the world hongry for what you denied it." Ruth could not bite enough. Her teeth were on edge with the yearning. Like the impulse of a cat to claw, she searched for crunchy things, and when there was nothing, she would grind her teeth. (pp. 131–32)
	Later, when Ruth is in a rage, she resumes cornstarch-eating.	She tasted again the Argo cornstarch and felt the marvelous biting and crunching it allowed her. (pp. 135–36)

White Is for Witching (Oyeyemi 2009)	The novel focuses on the relationship between fraternal twins, Miranda and Eliot. Miranda has pica, and it is central to the book; the title under which it was originally published in the UK was even *Pie-Kah*. There are many passages on pica (cf. pp. 3, 18, 20–22, 46, 52, 70, 150, and 175), including this one, narrated by her brother.	What Miri did was, she crammed chalk into her mouth under her covers. She hid the packaging at the bottom of her bag and threw it away when we got to school. But then there'd be cramps that twisted her body, pushed her off her seat and lay her on the floor, helplessly pedalling her legs. Once, as if she knew that I was thinking of sampling her chalk to see what the big wow was, she smiled sweetly, sadly, patronisingly and said to me, "Don't start, you'll get stuck." (p. 21)
Survivor: A Novel (Palahniuk 1999)	The narrator is one of a dwindling number of survivors of a religious cult in which most members have already killed themselves.	The girl last night, the only other remaining survivor of the Creedish church district, she ate dirt. There's even a name for it. They call it geophagy. This was popular among the Africans brought to America as slaves. Popular probably isn't the right word. (p. 170)
The Scowrers: A comedy (Shadwell 1691)	A bawdy latenight discourse on people's desires: alcohol, sex, and pica substances (For "Green-sickness," see *chlorosis* in glossary.)	Green-sickness Maids now dream of Clay and Lime For example, the thirsty Drunkard dreams of Bottle Ale, Or sucking a whole Barrel from the Tap; The Oyly Cookmaid stretches now, and yawns, And calls on *Dick* the Plowman in her Sleep, Who snores with Fumes from *Suffolk* Cheese and Bacon: Green-sickness Maids now dream of Clay and Lime. Now what a Devil's this to my business if they do? either begin your serenade, or I will roar and wake your Mistriss with my shrill melodious Pipe. (p. 43)
East of Eden (Steinbeck 2002 [1952])	Cathy is a conscienceless character who commits terrible crimes throughout her	She was misshapen; her belly, tight and heavy and distended, made it impossible for her to stand without supporting herself with her hands. . . . And a woman was likely to

life, including burning down her parents' house with them locked inside. She is said to represent Satan. This scene describes her pregnancy with twins.

have strange tastes, some said for filth, and it was set down to the Eve nature still under sentence for original sin.

Cathy's odd appetite was simple compared to some. The carpenters, repairing the old house, complained that they could not keep the lumps of chalk with which they coated their chalk lines. Again and again the scored hunks disappeared. Cathy stole them and broke them in little pieces. She carried the chips in her apron pocket, and when no one was about she crushed the soft lime between her teeth. She spoke very little. (pp. 184–85)

The Grapes of Wrath (Steinbeck 1967 [1939])

Rose of Sharon, pregnant and bereft of a husband, eats "slack lime" or calcium oxide. She eats it as she talks about how she wishes she had milk to drink, like the doctor told her she should.

"I see you nibblin' on somepin. What you eatin'?"
"Nothin'."
"Come on, what you nibblin' on?"
"Jus' a piece a slack lime. Foun' a big hunk."
"Why, tha's jus' like eatin' dirt."
"I kinda feel like I wan' it."
Ma was silent. She spread her knees and tightened her skirt. "I know," she said at last. "I et coal oncet when I was in a fambly way. Et a big piece a coal. Granma says I shouldn'." (p. 368)

Chronicles of Pineville (Thompson 1852)

Describing the cast of poor whites who frequented Mr. Harley's store to drink liquor on Saturdays, the author describes:

"those who allowed their mother earth to enter largely into their daily provender, of whom there were not a few in those days" (p. 40)

Fights regularly broke out among those with the habit of eating earth:

the torpid clay-eater, his bloated, watery countenance illuminated by the exhilarating qualities of rum, as he closed in with his antagonist, and showed by his performances that he could eat clay as well in its animate as in its inanimate form. (p. 41)

Eden (Vernon 2003)

The night before Maddie's invalid aunt, Aunt Pip, returns to the hospital for further treatment for breast cancer, Aunt Pip eats

When the clay began to break, she [Aunt Pip] picked up the pieces around her and ate them. With each lump, she looked behind her, as if something was there.
"Open your mouth," Aunt Pip said fearlessly. She had crushed the red dirt into

red clay that had caked
onto a glass lantern.
She then feeds Maddie
some.

a fine powder in the palm of her hand.
"Taste it."
    I did.
    This was God. It was different from the
cracker of Communion. It tasted of rain. The
rain that had fallen off the rooftops of every
house in Pyke County had formed a red river
of blood. You should have tasted this. I was
eating the brightest star in the sky. I was
swallowing the taste of God. (pp. 141–42)

Association Between Pica and Iron Deficiency and/or Anemia in Cross-Sectional Studies (n=28)[a]

Population	Location	N	Relationship between Pica, Anemia, and/or Iron Deficiency[b]	Prevalence of Pica[c]	Reference
Women attending antenatal clinics	Pemba Island, Tanzania	2,361	Any pica was associated with lower Hb (g/dL; multivariate model OR 0.76, CI: 0.72, 0.81)	Any: 40.1%; starch, 36.3%; earth, 5.2%	Young et al. 2010
HIV+ pregnant women enrolled in Vitamin A trial	Dar es Salaam, Tanzania	971	Geophagy was associated with an increased risk of anemia (adjusted RR 1.16; CI:0.98–1.36) and a lower Hb (adjusted-mean difference –0.38 g/dL; CI: –0.73, –0.04)	Earth: 29%	Antelman et al. 2000; Kawai et al. 2009
Recent parturients	Buenos Aires, Argentina	327	Women with any pica had significantly higher SF, EP, TSAT, and a greater proportion had IDA than matched controls	Any pica: 21.9%	Lopez et al. 2001; Lopez et al. 2007

Men and non-pregnant women from general population	Mwanza region, Tanzania	1,498	Adult geophagists had significantly lower SF and Hb in numerous multivariate models	Earth among women: 19%; among men, 4%	Malenganisho et al. 2007
Women attending antenatal clinics	New Halfa Teaching Hospital, Eastern Sudan	744	Geophagists were significantly more likely to be anemic (multivariate model OR 1.65, CI: 1.05, 2.6)	Not stated	Adam et al. 2005
School-children 7–15 y	Lusaka, Zambia	406	No SD in mean Hb at baseline by geophagy status	Earth among girls: 80.2%; among boys, 67.7%	Nchito et al. 2004
Women attending rural antenatal health clinics	North Carolina, USA	128	No SD in Hb or HCT by pica status	Any pica: 38%; ice: 36.7%; starch, 4.7%; earth, 1.6%	Corbett et al. 2003
Healthy women attending antenatal clinics, 16 w gestational age	Shiraz, Iran	270	No SD in SF by geophagy status	Earth: 28.3%	Karimi et al. 2002
Women attending 4 antenatal clinics	Accra, Ghana	502	Mean Hb throughout pregnancy among geophagists was 0.81 g/dL lower than non-geophagists	Earth: 28.5%; starch, 3.6%; chalk, 1.2%	Tayie and Lartey 1999
Participants in WIC program	Houston and Prairie View, Tex., USA	281	Women with pica had 0.4 to 0.8 g/dL lower Hb at birth than women without pica	Any pica: 76.5%; ice/frost, 68.3%; other, 8.2%	Rainville 1998

Women attending antenatal clinics	Kilfi District Hospital, Coastal Kenya	275	Geophagists had lower Hb (9.1 vs.10.0 g/dL) and SF (4.5 vs. 9.0 µg/L) than non-geophagists	Earth: 56%	Geissler et al. 1998b
Random sample of children 10–18 y	Western Kenya	156	Proportion of anemic (Hb < 11.0 g/dl) and of Fe-depleted (SF < 12 µg/l) children was higher among geophageous children (9.6% vs. 0% anemic; 18.4% vs. 5.4% Fe-depleted)	Earth: 73.1%	Geissler et al. 1998a
Women attending antenatal clinics	Katima Mulilo clinic, Eastern Caprivi, Namibia	171	Geophagists more likely to be anemic (multivariate model OR 2.99, CI: 1.52, 5.86)	Earth: 44.4%	Thomson 1997
Women attending antenatal clinics	Muscogee County, Ga., USA	125	No SD in % anemic between those who engaged in pica and those who did not	Any pica: 14.4%; ice, 6.4%; earth, 4%; starch, 4%; other, 6.4%	Smulian et al. 1995
Pregnant women 13–24 y	Camden, N.J., USA	1,334	Pagophagists and those with other picas had significantly lower SF, folate, and plasma Zn at 28 w gestation than those without pica	Ice: 53%; other (predominantly starch), 7%	Coles et al. 1995
Women 16–35 y at antenatal clinics and hospitals	Washington, D.C., USA	553	SF (15.6 ng/mL vs. 27.1) and MC Hb (29.5 pg vs. 30.8) were significantly lower among women with pica	Any pica (ice, frost, starch, other): 8.1%	Edwards et al. 1994

Recent parturients	Atlanta, Ga., USA	109	No SD between recalled anemia and recalled pica behavior	Ice: 18.3%; earth, 2.7%; starch, 2.7%; other, 1%	Kirsch 1990
WIC clients	Pitt County, N.C., USA	190	People with IDA 8.4 times more likely to engage in pica	Any pica: 34.7%; starch, 22.1; earth, 7.4; ice, 5.3	Butler 1982
City health department antenatal clinics	Houston, Tex., USA	47	No SD in HCT or proportion anemic between pagophagists and non-pagophagists	Not determined	Speer 1980
Women in active labor at Cook County Hospital	Chicago, Ill., USA	623	Anemia twice as frequent among starch eaters	Starch: 24.4%	Keith et al. 1975
Black population, pregnancy status not clear	Rural Holmes County, Miss., USA	500 HH with 368 anemic women	No difference in HCT by pica status	Earth among pregnant and postpartum women: 28%; other pica, 19%	Frate 1984; Vermeer and Frate 1975; Vermeer and Frate 1979
Consecutive patients at antenatal clinics	Georgia, USA	410	Mean serum Fe in women with pica 60.1µg/100mL vs. 98.5 µg/100mL in controls	Any pica (starch, chalk, clay): 16%	Bronstein and Dollar 1974
Women in active labor at Cook County Hospital	Chicago, Ill., USA	987	Hb 9.6 g/dL in amylophagists vs. 10.2 g/dL in non-amylophagists; HCT 35.2 in amylophagists vs. 34.0; 13.2% of amylophagists had Hb < 8.0g/dL vs. 8.1%	Starch: 34.6%	Keith et al. 1968

Randomly selected postnatal inpatients	Urban and rural areas of Augusta, Ga., USA	200	No SD in Hb between pica and non-pica groups at initial antenatal visit or delivery	Any pica: 55%; earth, 32.5%; starch, 19%; other, 3.5%	O'Rourke et al. 1967
Antenatal clinic attendees	Tuskegee Institute, Ala., USA	62	27% of clay-eaters, 17% of cornstarch eaters, and 7% of non-pica group had Hb <10 g/dL	Not stated	Edwards et al. 1964
Consecutive pregnant women	Philadelphia, Pa., USA	50	No SD in Hb by amylophagy	Starch: 26%	Sage 1962
Married women 20–30 y attending antenatal clinics	New York, N.Y., USA	275	Hb among 100 women with pica 11.07g/dL vs. 11.2 g/dL among women with no pica	Any pica (starch, clay, other): 42.9%	Dunston 1961
Children 2–5 y old	Washington, D.C.	30 cases with pica, 28 matched controls	Children with pica had significantly lower Hb than children with no pica (10.1 g/dL +1.36 vs. 11.2 g/dL +1.02); P < 0.01)	Purposively selected population	Gutelius et al. 1962

[a] *Abbreviations:* CI—95% Confidence interval, EP—Erythrocyte Porphyrin, Hb—hemoglobin concentration, HCT—Hematocrit, IDA—iron deficiency anemia, m—month, MC Hb—Mean corpuscular hemoglobin, HH—household, OR—odds ratio, RR—relative risk, SD—significant difference, TSAT—transferrin saturation, w—week, y—year
[b] Shaded cells indicate studies in which significant differences in iron status were found.
[c] All reported values statistically significant at $p < 0.05$

Association Between Pica and Zinc Deficiency in Cross-Sectional Studies (n=6)[a]

Population	Location	N	Relationship of Pica to Zn Status[b]	Reference
Children between 18 m and 48 m	Chandigarh, northern India	31 cases with pica, 60 matched controls	Mean plasma Zn level in the pica group (60 µg/dL) lower than that of controls (110.2 µg/dL)	Singhi et al. 2003
Institutionalized adults with mental retardation	North Carolina, USA	128 residents with pica, 30 controls	54% of the pica group were found to have a low Zn level, falling below 0.90 µg/dL vs. 7% of the controls	Lofts et al. 1990
Turkish 3–24 y	Turkey	Not stated	Zn in serum, RBC, hair and urine was significantly lower in those with geophagy compared to controls	Cavdar et al. 1983
Indian children 9 m to 7 y	India	20 cases with pica, 22 controls	Serum Zn was lower in those with pica (72.5 µg /dL) vs. controls	Bhalla et al. 1983

			(117.7 µg/ dL); a greater proportion with pica were anemic (75%) vs. controls (27%)	
Institutionalized mentally retarded adults	Not stated	60 cases with pica, 6 controls	Plasma Zn was lower in people with pica (67 µg/dL) vs. those without (82 µg/dL)	Danford et al. 1982
Children 5–21 y	Turkey	32 cases of geophagy, 20 controls	Serum, hair, and urine Zn were all significantly lower in geophagists	Cavdar et al. 1980

[a] *Abbreviations:* m—month, RBC—red blood cells, y—year
[b] Shaded cells indicate studies in which significant differences in iron status were found, all reported values statistically significant at p < 0.05.

Predictions

HUNGER HYPOTHESIS

Prediction 1. People eating non-food substances have little other food to eat.

Prediction 2. People would feel less hungry after eating pica substances.

Prediction 3. Pica substances would not be desired when "typical" food was available.

Prediction 4. Almost any non-food item would be eaten by the consumer.

MICRONUTRIENT HYPOTHESIS

Prediction 5. Pica would be associated with a micronutrient deficiency populations with the highest micronutrient needs.

Prediction 6. Pica would be associated with populations with the highest micronutrient requirements.

Prediction 7. Elimination of the deficiency would cause pica to cease.

Prediction 8. Pica substances would provide micronutrients in which the consumer is deficient.

PROTECTION HYPOTHESIS

Prediction 9. Pica substances would shield us from the harmful effects of toxins and pathogens.

Prediction 10. Pica would occur more frequently during exposure to toxins and pathogens.

Prediction 11. Pica would occur more frequently when people are vulnerable to the harmful effects of toxins and pathogens.

Notes

1. What on Earth?

1. The term *pica* has many meanings outside the context of non-food cravings. The Pica were a gang in West Side Chicago in the 1960s (Suttles 1968) and in a Bosnian Muslim village in the early 1980s, pica was slang for the vagina of a virgin (Lockwood 1983). PICA was the Palestine Jewish Colonization Association and still is a pseudoaneurysm of the internal carotid artery.

2. Geophagy has by far the most synonyms: aarde-eten, clay-eating, chalk-eating, dirt-eating, erde-essen, geomania, geophagia, géophagie, and jordæden.

3. Other "–phagies" found among nonhuman animals and extremely rarely among humans include coprophagy (feces), lithophagy (stones), trichophagy (hair or wool), and xylophagy (wood). Linguists with spare time have expanded the pica "–phagies" to substances far less frequently consumed, e.g., cautopyreiophagia (burnt matches) (Perry 1977) and geomelophagia (raw potatoes) (Johnson and Stephens 1982).

4. At an archaeolgical site at Kalambo Falls, Zambia, the bones of *Homo habilis* have been found together with white clay. Several facts suggest geophagy (Root-Bernstein and Root-Bernstein 1997). For one, the site predates any known use of clay for pottery or ornaments by tens of thousands of years, and the clay is not found naturally in the area, suggesting that it was carried there for a certain purpose. More intriguingly, it is similar to that which is presently consumed today by geophagists around the world.

5. It is possible that this smell is due to geosmin, an organic compound with a distinctly earthy smell (Gerber and Lechevalier 1965).

6. Cooking starches breaks down large starch molecules into simple sugars that are more easily digested. Without exposure to heat, most ingested starches pass out of our bodies without being metabolized.

7. Although they probably don't know it, these women were following centuries-old advice from Roman (Oribasius et al. 1851, bk. 5, p. 197) and Byzantine (Aetius of Amida/Ricci 1542 [1950]; Paulus Aegineta and Adams 1844, bk. 1, sec. 1) physicians, who suggested that starch be given instead of earth to geophagic women.

8. Cornstarch is made by extracting the starch from the corn kernel under high pressure and heat, which makes the carbohydrates in it digestible, i.e., many calories are available.

9. On the Yahoo! Cornstarch mailing list, one amylophagist recently suggested that microwaving powderized Argo starch can return it to chunk form.

2. A Biocultural Approach

1. A more expansive treatment of the concept *biocultural* is outside the scope of this book. For further reading on it, see Goodman and Leatherman (1998), Pelto et al. (2000), Roth (2004), and Wiley (1992).

2. The primary references used throughout the book can roughly be classified into seven categories:

1. Individual case reports: "a Turkish woman living in Paris ate chalk and clay every day" (Henon et al. 1975).

2. An enumerated population: "55% of anemic Namibian women eat earth" (Thomson 1997).

3. A cultural group: "pregnant Otomacs regularly engage in clay-eating (von Humboldt et al. 1821).

4. Animal studies: "African buffalo frequently engage in geophagic behavior on Mount Kenya" (Mahaney 1987).

5. Soil analysis studies: "montmorillonite was major component of ch'aqu" (Browman and Gunderson 1993).

6. Literature reviews in which no new data were presented: "According to Labilladiere and confirmed by the reports of Hekmeyer [clay] figures are crunched on by women and children" (Ferrand 1886).

7. Experimental studies, such as a randomized clinical study in which micronutrients are given and changes in pica behavior are measured (Nchito et al. 2004).

3. There have been some very ambiguous, and therefore useless, definitions set forth by physicians: "the eating of any foreign substance" (Halsted 1968) and "the

compulsive eating of anything" (Crosby 1976b). More specific, and therefore more valuable, definitions of pica in scientific communities include "the persistent eating of non-nutritive substances" (World Health Organization 1993) and "the tendency or craving to eat substances other than normal foodstuffs" (2000). But even these definitions have serious limitations. The term *non-nutritive* is problematic because nutrients *can* be obtained from some pica substances. Some starches are high in calories, and it is possible that micronutrients can be obtained from some soils. The phrase "normal foodstuffs" is ambiguous because normalcy is distinctly culturally determined. For example, one could argue that uncooked rice is nearly food, it's just raw food, and that cornstarch is an ingredient used in the preparation of foods. Zanzibaris group the consumption of unripe mangoes with geophagy and amylophagy, but in much of Asia, unripe mangoes are a regular snack (Young and Pelto 2006). Therefore, a definition that considers what the *consumer* regards as normal food is more useful because it recognizes the variation in ethnotaxonomies of food. Finally, both of these definitions fall short because neither mentions the strong desires that are a hallmark of pica.

4. The phrase "ultimate explanation" has irked many who study proximate explanations. It's not meant to suggest one is more important than the other, only to distinguish immediate causes from long-term causes.

5. The hypotheses most worth exploring are hunger (chapter 7), micronutrient deficiency (chapter 8), and protection (chapter 9). There are two other adaptive hypotheses about the etiology of pica that I do not explore at length in this book because they seem fairly implausible: stress and inoculation.

It has been suggested that pica is a "protective" response to stress, similar to nail-biting or smoking (Edwards et al. 1994; Solyom et al. 1991). However, there is minimal evidence to support this. In a study of 553 black women in Washington, D.C., pica was more frequent among those with less social support (Edwards et al. 1994), which was the basis for a rather vague conclusion that during pregnancy "pica may be a mediator of stress, acting through the immune system" (961s). Besides being insufficiently explicit about the mechanism by which pica substances would interact with the immune system, the manifestation of stress in the consumption of starch or ice (as opposed to other stress responses measured in the study, such as street drug use) is not adequately explained.

Pica, especially geophagy, has also been suggested to function as a type of inoculation; by consuming live microorganisms in soil, a pregnant woman will endow her fetus with immunity to those through the antigens she produces (Callahan 2003). The organic part of soil, the humus, contains a vast array of microbes; many of the antibiotics we use today have been grown from those found in soil. However, there are two reasons why geophagy is unlikely to serve as an inoculation. Geophagists choose soils that have low humus content; they mostly opt for clay-rich earths where there is less microbial activity. Second, it is unlikely that many microorganisms will survive the drying or baking typically done to prepare geophagic soils (cf. chapter 1). Furthermore, most antigens that a fetus needs will be created through the mother's everyday contact with harmful substances without necessitating her purposive ingestion of large quantities of soil or other non-food substances. Finally, this hypothesis does not explain non-geophagic pica.

6. Initially we searched online databases (Pubmed, JSTOR, OCLC, ISI Web of Science, Agricola, Dissertation Abstracts, Google Scholar, Human Relation Area Files, Library of Congress, LexisNexis, Proquest Historical Newspapers) for entries containing "aarde eten," "cachexia Africana," "chalk eating," "citta," "clay eating," "dirt eating," "erde essen," "geophagia," "geophagy," "mal d'estomac," "malacia," and "pica." We then used the reference lists of each publication to identify additional primary sources. This process was iterated until no new references were found. Our search was not restricted by language or date, so the database includes articles in many languages and spanning nearly 500 years.

7. The seven categories of life stages are as follows: (1) "preadolescents" are children who have not reached puberty (3–12 years old), (2) "adolescents" are boys and girls who have reached puberty (13–18 years old), (3) "pregnant women" are adolescent or adult women who are gestating, (4) "lactating women" are those who are breastfeeding, (5) "women" are adults whose pregnancy or lactation status is unknown, (6) "men" are adult males, and (7) "elderly" are those described in reports as being "old" or no longer bearing children.

8. The primary investigators of the large study were Drs. Rebecca Stoltzfus (Cornell University) and James Tielsch (Johns Hopkins). More on the study design and protocol can be found in Farag et al. (2007) and Young et al. (2010a, 2010b).

3. Medicine You Can Walk On

1. **Adsorption** and **absorption** are similar but not synonymous. *Adsorption* refers to the gathering molecules on a surface (think static cling on a cheap synthetic blouse). *Absorption* refers to the permeation of molecules (think a sponge saturated in water).

2. One beneficiary of the beautifying effects of clay was Cleopatra. She took mud baths regularly, and their beautifying consequences are alleged to have helped her to seduce not one but two of the most powerful men of her time, Julius Caesar and Mark Antony. This, in turn, helped her to achieve influential positions in a succession of Egyptian and Roman governments.

3. On a related note, a non-clay but still very finely powdered chalky substance called **diatomaceous earth** (because it is made of tiny fossilized diatoms) is also useful against insects, including those foot soldiers of urban ickiness, cockroaches.

4. Further elaboration on the events described in this section can be found in Dannenfeldt (1984), Hall and Photos-Jones (2008), Hasluck (1909), and Thompson (1914).

5. Dioscorides, a Greek physician and pharmacologist (40–90 A.D.), and his Roman contemporary Pliny the Elder, naturalist and military leader (23–79 A.D.), were

the first to write about the medical properties of terra sigillata. For some context, this was a time when all that was known about medicine, plants, agriculture, architecture, sculpture, geology, and mineralogy could be contained in one place: Pliny's book *Naturalis Historia*. Dioscorides was so knowledgeable (or, rather, scientific knowledge was so limited for so long) that his five-volume oeuvre, *De Materia Medica*, was the basis of most medical practice for 1,600 years (Dioscorides et al. 1934).

6. And even then, it nearly did not happen. On Galen's first attempt, on the way to Rome from Asia, the port at which they docked was on the opposite end of the island from the site of the terra sigillata, and the captain would not wait for the esteemed Galen to collect his specimens. On his second visit to Lemnos, on the way back home to Asia, Galen made sure to arrive at a port near the healing earth (Tozer 1890).

7. There are many accounts of such visits, but this is my favorite title: *The totall discourse of the rare adventures & painefull peregrinations of long nineteene yeares travayles from Scotland to the most famous kingdomes in Europe, Asia and Affrica* (Lithgow 1632).

8. The loss of female power accompanies many societies' conversion to monotheism. As Tom Robbins puts it, Christianity is "a system for turning priestesses into handmaidens, queens into concubines, and goddesses into muses" (Robbins 1984:51).

9. This antidiarrheal medicine, called *mustachoma*, is made of clay and grape juice boiled to a syrupy consistency.

10. In the 1980s, Kaopectate's manufacturers switched the active ingredient from kaolin to palygorskite, a clay with similar absorbent properties. In 1993 the formula was again changed, due to a lawsuit by the State of California contending that the lead levels in palygorskite were dangerous. This time, bismuth subsalicylate, the same active ingredient in Pepto-Bismol, replaced palygorskite, rendering "Kaopectate" a misnomer. These days, if you want clay in your Kaopectate, you need to go to Canada.

Clays do continue to be sold in other over-the-counter and prescription antidiarrheal medicines: Diarrest, Di-gon II, Diatrol, Donnagel, Kaopek, K-Pek, Parepectolin, and Smecta. Most of these are not available in the United States.

11. Veterinarians used to recommend that pet owners use Kaopectate to treat their pets' diarrhea, but because bismuth subsalicylate is an aspirin derivative, Kaopectate is no longer safe to feed to your furry friend. Palygorskite is, however, available in the United States for animal consumption in a product called Dia-sorb.

12. Smecta™ is rarely used in the United States, for reasons I do not understand.

13. Much of the information in the rest of this section is drawn from Reinbacher (2002).

14. Clays have, however, been used in various health movements (e.g., Knishinsky 1998; Post-Dispatch 1902). For example, in 1902, seventy-five men and women were persuaded by St. Louis resident William Windsor to eat a daily dose of earth

(Post-Dispatch 1902). From the journalist's description, Windsor sounds like an endearing armchair scientist. "Kris Kringle himself is not a more rotund nor more rollicking character than Dirt Eater Windsor. . . . He can sit in a chair and tweedle his thumbs on his stomach, which they say is the pièce de résistance in happiness." Windsor explained his decision to become a geophagist. "I wondered why men were not as healthy as animals. I observed that almost every man had stomach troubles and that the wild animals had good stomachs. I became convinced that their good health was due to the fact that they were dirt eaters." He then tried it and experienced "such great success" that he began teaching dirt-eating. The dirt he and his adherents ate came from river bottoms, and was sterilized and distributed at a cost of about 10 cents/week (approximately $2.50 in 2010). He carried a sack with him wherever he went, and clearly relished it. During the interview, he took a heaping spoonful and "swallow[ed] it with that sly wink with which a Kentucky colonel takes his whiskey. He [sent] a glass of water to chase it, and heaves a huge sigh of content."

4. Religious Geophagy

1. The three were fleeing to Egypt because King Herod, fearing he would eventually be usurped by the then-newborn Jesus, had called for the slaughter of all boys under the age of two.

2. Another extraordinary property of this grotto is its power to unify religious faiths. It is a sanctuary venerated by both Christians and Muslims, reflected by the Roman and Arabic script found throughout. It's lovely to find common ground in an era of so much Christian-Muslim animosity.

3. There is plenty of evidence of influence of Mayan culture on the Cult of the Black Christ in Esquipulas; most prominent is the crucifix that is the centerpiece of the Basilica. The first crucifix was made by a famous Portuguese craftsman, Quirio Cataño, and was installed in the chapel in 1595. According to one Equipulas scholar, darker balsam wood was chosen for the crucifix "because the Indians, terrified by the cruelty of the Spaniards, believed that all white men were evil and that Christ could not be a kind and charitable god if he were white" (Kelsey and Osborne 1939). The cross is decorated with a carved vine and golden leaves that resemble the Tree of Life, an important symbol in Mayan culture. The already dark-complected statue slowly blackened from the smoke of candles and incense at Christ's bleeding feet, until it became deep black it is today. The black color of the statue may have also helped the statue of Christ fit into the local cosmology because of the power of the color black in Mayan and Aztec cultures (De Borhegyi 1954). Because of Esquipulas, eating benditos is almost invariably connected with the worship of a miraculous Black Christ. However, this is only in the Americas; Black Christ images in Europe and Africa are not associated with geophagy.

4. Geophagy was by no means unique to Esquipulas. A number of observers of indigenous culture during the early days of Spanish colonialism wrote about how the thick cakes made of earth, sand, and slimy substances from the surface of Lake Texcoco were eaten (e.g., Torquemada 1723; Diaz del Castillo et al. 1908; López de Gomara 1554).

5. To understand Don Abeyta, a bit of Catholic history is in order. St. Francis of Assisi recognized three religious orders important to the Roman Catholic community. Friars and brothers were the first order, cloistered nuns were the second, and the third was laity in the community, the Brothers and Sisters of Penance. Los Hermanos de la Fraternidad Piadosa de Nuestro Padre Jesús Nazareno (Los Hermanos Penitentes, for short) is one of hundreds of groups belonging to the third order. Los Hermanos Penitentes believe that sin can only be atoned for by suffering, and suffering in this sect has taken the form of excruciating practices: whipping oneself in the same place with a knot of cactus; dragging heavy crosses up rocky mountains using ropes that cut deep grooves into the flesh; and maintaining open wounds (crucifix-shaped, on the back) for the forty days of Lent (Prince 1915). The Penitentes were critical to the survival of Catholicism because they performed many of the religious rites for which there were not enough priests. Plus, they are very important to this part of New Mexico since one of their brethren helped to found Chimayo.

6. El Posito is refilled regularly by the parish priest, who buys 25 tons of earth every year (Sharlet 2002).

7. Maria Martinez, a potter who made the black-on-black San Ildefonso pottery famous, was one of these pilgrims (Marriott 1948). As a child, she fell very sick. Her mother made a promise to God that if Maria survived, they would walk to Chimayo. During her pilgrimage, at age 10, her mother directed her to rub her body down with the earth from El Posito as well as to collect a jarful of it, to later mix with water and drink while reciting Our Father. A number of pages of her biography are devoted to her experiences at Chimayo (see Appendix D for more on this passage).

8. The same Karbala where suicide bombers continue to kill and maim hundreds today, especially on holy days associated with Imam Hussein.

9. Graveyard earth has been used outside of hoodoo, e.g., in nineteenth-century Ireland, people would "take the clay or mold from the graves of priests and boil it with milk as a decoction for the cure of disease" (Gomme 1892:114).

10. In fact, hoodoo offers a number of exquisite punishments for your better half. For example, a woman can cause her husband to become bent at the waist for months and months by burying a bottle filled with "his skin, his urine and his action [ahem!] and everything" (Hyatt 1970:430).

11. For more information about hoodoo, Catherine Yronwode's Lucky Mojo Web site (luckymojo.com) is an excellent resource. And if you really want to learn a lot more about hoodoo, you can take her "Hoodoo Magic Spells Correspondence Course."

5. Poisons and Pathogens

1. Cutoffs for the definitions of mild, moderate, and severe anemia vary by sex and age (Stoltzfus and Dreyfuss 1998). In pregnant women, for example, hemoglobin concentration lower than 11.0 g/dL is considered anemic, and hemoglobin lower than 7.0 g/dL is considered severely anemic.

2. In 1922, General Motors researchers discovered that adding tetraethyl lead to gasoline reduced engine knock, allowing development of large, powerful automobiles with high-compression engines. At the time, public health experts, government officials, scientists, and corporate leaders were aware of the dangers posed by the introduction of lead into gasoline (Rosner and Markowitz 1985). Nevertheless, in the 1920s, DuPont, GM, and Standard Oil promoted the addition of tetraethyl lead to gasoline, with the aid of a sexy mechanic, Ethyl. "Take me with you and get a kick out of driving," she urged drivers. These companies argued that leaded gasoline was essential to the industrial progress of America. Even the fact that, in 1924, 80% of Standard Oil's forty-nine tetraethyl lead plant workers died or were severely poisoned from organic lead did not slow progress; the company attributed these injuries to worker carelessness (Rosner and Markowitz 1985).

3. All of these instances involve people without any known mental problems. Individuals with mental illness or developmental disorders are much more likely to ingest overtly toxic substances. In these populations there have been reports of compulsive ingestion of coins and other small metal objects (François and Brenet 2004; Hasan et al. 1995; Hassan et al. 2000), feces (Beck and Frohberg 2005), and even disposable lighters (Dean et al. 2004). This is discussed in chapter 6.

4. All primates, not just humans, host geohelminths, as do some smaller mammals.

6. Dismissal and Damnation

1. Not that the crud in the dustpan is what people are seeking out anyway, but to a non-geophagist, dirt may appear to be created equally.

2. From the New International Version:

Psalm 72.9: The desert tribes will bow before him and his enemies will lick the dust.

Isaiah 49.23: Kings will be your foster fathers, and their queens your nursing mothers. They will bow down before you with their faces to the ground; they will lick the dust at your feet. Then you will know that I am the Lord; those who hope in me will not be disappointed.

Micah 7.17: They will lick dust like a snake, like creatures that crawl on the ground. They will come trembling out of their dens; they will turn in fear to the Lord our God and will be afraid of you.

3. However, in the last century, pica is more frequently reported among black women than among any other demographic in the United States.

4. It is clear from physicians' descriptions of pica that for many of them their sympathies rested with slave owners, e.g., "Persons with indulgent masters and owners, who are themselves the real slaves, while the owned are only *nominally* so, provided with food, raiment, and, if necessary, medical aid, are the subject of this malady" (Cragin 1835:361).

5. For further reading on the use of masks among slaves, see Handler and Steiner (2006) and MacClancy (2007).

6. I might add this highly simplistic understanding of pregnancy was based on a scene from *Lady and the Tramp* in which Jim Dear's pregnant wife (Lady's "mother") sends him out in a winter storm to get chop suey and ice cream. All he can do is "yes, dear" her, shaking his head at his wife's misguided palate.

7. Today, both the geophagic and nasty connotations of these nicknames have faded, such that *Sandlappers* is the name of South Carolina's state magazine, choral groups, elementary schools, and a song sung by schoolchildren (Welch 2008).

8. I can't resist the inclusion of another of Davenport's great culinary moments: "A weekend away from paratrooper barracks when we dined on eggs scrambled in Jack Daniel's, potato chips, and peanut brittle, while the Sergeant Major, a family man of bankerish decorum in ordinary times, sang falsetto 'There Will Be Peace in the Valley' stark naked except for cowboy boots and hat" (Davenport 1980:137).

8. Pica as a Micronutrient Supplement

1. For greater scientific detail than what is presented in this chapter, see Young (2010).

2. "After a few Weeks time she would rejoyce more to see a Shoulder of Mutton well roasted, than a Handful of Mortar out of the Wall, or a Plate of Oatmeal, the usual Viands she formerly delighted in" (Peirce 1697:193–94).

3. *Anemia* was not a term that was in use for most of the time period encompassed by the Pica Literature Database, but *chlorosis* was; it is now considered to be synonymous with anemia (Hudson 1977).

4. Such differences in hemoglobin concentration were clearly driven by iron deficiency, as indicated by measures of zinc protoporphyrin.

5. Infants' ingestion of earth is not readily defined as pica because it's difficult to determine as purposive, or not.

6. People took Avicenna's medical writings very seriously; his 14-volume masterpiece, the *Canon of Medicine*, was the main textbook for medical education up until the seventeenth century.

7. For example, in Kenya the Luo preferred the white clay sold at the market to the reddish clay that could be collected locally (Geissler 2000). Vermeer reported that iron was removed from geophagic clays by Ewe people in Ghana (Vermeer

1971). In Alabama, red clay was eaten, but white was preferred because it was "less gritty" (Spencer 2002).

8. I.e., adding 50 mL of 0.1 N HCl to 5 g of soil and then shaking it for 30 minutes.

9. The removal of calcium from the soil caused other trace elements to become concentrated, and so the contribution of zinc may be overestimated.

10. Their association could be explained by the following scenario: anemia is a response to inflammation; the body sequesters iron in storage such that it is not available for invading pathogens. Pica may also be a response to inflammation (cf. chapter 9). Thus, they may be correlated, but not causally linked.

11. Micronutrient deficiencies may serve an adapative purpose in some settings.

9. Pica to Protect and Detoxify

1. Today we face fewer plant secondary compounds than we did even a few centuries ago. They have mostly been bred out of many of the crops that we eat through the process of domestication (although some compounds, like caffeine, which is an alkaloid, have been selectively bred for).

2. These are described in greater detail in Young (2010). One of the cleanest studies of the capacity of kaolin to bind plant secondary compounds was conducted by Dominy and colleagues (2004). They used a TNO intestinal model, a kind of sophisticated chitty-chitty bang-bang contraption with four successive silicon tubing compartments that simulate digestion, right down to peristalsis (contractions of the intestines that move food forward). They placed 300 g test meals with four different plant toxins into the TNO model with and without 10 g of purified kaolin. Clay adsorbed approximately 30% of toxins. And because there was no mucosal layer on the silicon tubing, there could be no residual clay hanging around as there likely is in the intestines of a geophagist, so this was likely an underestimate of the detoxification capacity of kaolin in a living organism.

3. It was only in the early 1970s that Hladik and Gueguen first proposed that geophagy was protective against toxins consumed by primates (1974). Fourteen years later, in 1988, Profet first suggested that clays could be protective against human teratogens (chemicals, microbes, radiation, etc. that harm the fetus) (Profet 1992). Colleagues and I suggested the potential for non-earth pica substances to detoxify and protect only recently (Young et al. 2008; S. L. Young, P. W. Sherman, J. B. Lucks, and G. H. Pelto, unpublished observations).

4. Gilardi and colleagues (1999) studied the composition of the soil consumed (the type of clay, if any, and the presence of any elements), its capacity to change pH (also known as the buffering capacity), and its toxin adsorption capacity, both under in vitro and in vivo conditions. With these data, they were also able to test hypotheses about geophagy being motivated by parrots' need for grit (toothless par-

rots need help to grind up food), to change the pH of the gut, and to supply micro-nutrients. None of these were supported.

5. Hemoperfusion is similar to hemodialysis, except blood is passed through a column containing an adsorbent substance, which in this case was charcoal and clay (Lotan et al. 1983).

6. Analysis of the distribution of other picas by climate type has yet to be performed.

7. In Pemba, we found that there was more pica in later pregnancy, which is the opposite of what this hypothesis predicts. This may be explained by recall bias—most women were asked questions about their pica only at the end of their pregnancy, by which time they may have forgotten about their early tastes for earth and starch (see story of Mama Hamisa's forgetfulness under "Concealment of Pica Today," in chapter 6).

Glossary

Adaptation: genetic, physiological, or sociocultural adjustments to meet material needs in response to ecological challenges.

Absorption: the permeation of molecules into a substance, e.g., a sponge saturated with water.

Activated charcoal: charcoal that has been processed with steam at very high temperatures, making it extremely porous and thus giving it a very large surface area.

Adaptive: term used to describe behavior that contributes directly or indirectly to an individual's survival or reproductive success in a given ecological niche; opposite of nonadaptive.

Adsorption: the gathering of molecules on a surface, e.g., static cling on a cheap synthetic blouse.

Anemia: the condition of having too low of hemoglobin concentration. This could be caused by blood loss or insufficient red blood cell production due to inadequate dietary intake, infectious causes, or genetics.

Amylophagy: the purposive consumption of raw starch.

Benditos: sacred earth, also referred to as *panecitos, pan del señor,* and *tierra santa.*

Bioavailable: degree to which a nutrient is available to a target organ or tissue.

Cation: a negatively charged atom, i.e., the number of electrons is greater than the number of protons. Examples of cations include Fe^{3+}, Fe^{2+}, Mg^{2+}, and K^+.

Cation exchange capacity (CEC): a measure of how readily a substance can exchange adsorbed cations with cations in a surrounding solution.

Chlorosis: literally, "green sickness" and an antiquated term considered to be a synonym for *anemia*.

Clay: the finest inorganic component of soils, < 0.002 mm.

Clay minerals: Term used to refer to groups of clays with similar layer structures; examples include illite, montmorillonite, and smectite.

Confounder: term in epidemiology that refers to a phenomenon that affects both cause and effect, e.g., inflammation in the relationship between anemia and pica.

Diatomaceous earth: a soft, crumbly, porous sedimentary deposit formed from the fossil remains of diatoms; also known as kieselguhr.

Effect modification: term in epidemiology that refers to a phenomenon that modifies the strength of the relationship between cause X and outcome Y. For example, speeding (X) can cause a car accident (Y), but being drunk (the effect modifier) while speeding greatly increases the likelihood of a car accident.

Geohelminth: parasitic nematodes transmitted by soil. Examples include roundworms (*Ascaris lumbricoides*), whipworms (*Trichuris trichuria*), and hookworms (*Ancylostoma duodenale* and *Necator americanus*).

Geophagy: the purposive consumption of earth.

Glossitis: inflammation of the tongue.

Heme iron: one of two forms of dietary iron. Heme iron, which is only found in animal source foods, is iron that has already been integrated into cells and is therefore more bioavailable than inorganic, or non-heme, iron.

Hemoglobin (Hb): a protein responsible for transporting oxygen in the blood of vertebrates. Its molecule comprises four subunits, each containing an iron atom bound to a heme group. In pregnant women, hemoglobin concentration lower than 11.0 g/dL is considered anemic, and hemoglobin lower than 7.0 g/dL is considered severely anemic.

Hemoglobinopathy: gene mutation that results in abnormal structure of hemoglobin, e.g., sickle-cell disease, thalassemia.

Humus: One of the four components of soil (the others are sand, clay, and silt). It is the rich, dark organic material in soils and the site of most organic activity.

In vitro: studies done outside of a living organism, e.g., in a test tube or petri dish (from the Latin, "in glass").

In vivo: studies done in a living organism (from the Latin, "in a living thing").

Kaolin: one of the clay mineral groups (see table 3.1, p. 34).

Kaolinite: a particular species of clay that belongs to the kaolin family (see table 3.1, p. 34). Historically referred to as bolus alba.

Köppen climate classification system: One of the most widely used climate classification systems, it establishes criteria by which areas of the world could be categorized by climates, based on vegetation, temperature, and amount and seasonality of precipitation. It was created by Russian climatologist Vladimir Köppen in 1884.

Micronutrient: a chemical element or substance required in trace amounts for the normal growth and development of living organisms.

Null hypothesis: the hypothesis that there is no significant difference between specified populations.

P-value: the probability of obtaining a test statistic at least as extreme as the one that was actually observed. Most scientists use a p-value of 0.05 as a cutoff for calling a finding significant.

Pagophagy: The purposive consumption of large quantities of ice.

pH: a value that indicates the acidity or alkalinity of a solution on a logarithmic scale. The range is 1–14; the lower the number the greater the acidity. Gastric pH is fairly acidic, around 2; intestinal pH is nearly neutral, around 7.

Pica: the craving and purposive consumption of items that the consumer does not consider to be food for more than a month. Other terms for this behavior include cachexia, cachexia Africana, chthonophagia, hapsicoria, mal d'estomac, malacia, and paroroexia.

Radio-labeling: the incorporation of a radioactive tracer into a substance to be able to follow its activity.

Secondary compounds: toxic chemicals produced by plants to protect themselves from predation and infection. Examples include alkaloids, phenolics, saponins, tannins, and terpenes.

Standard Cross-Cultural Sample: A representative sample of 186 relatively independent cultures used by scholars who engage in cross-cultural research. It was created by George Murdock and Douglas White in 1969.

Terra sigillata: small clay tablets "stamped" or "sealed" with an insignia indicating their origin (see chapter 3).

Tinbergen's Four Questions: Four categories of explanations of animal behavior, including causation (mechanisms), development (ontogeny), evolutionary origins (phylogeny), and functional consequences.

Trimester: A period of three months. Pregnancies are often discussed in terms of first, second, and third trimesters.

Works Cited

1846. Un ésclave marron, au Brésil. *Le Magasin Pittoresque* 14: 229.

1866 (Apr. 7). From the South: Southern journeyings and jottings. *New York Times.*

1873. News and miscellany. *Medical and Surgical Reporter* 29: 417.

1897. The clay eaters. *Scientific American* 76: 150.

1967. An urge for Argo. *Time* 90: 36–37.

1969. Pica and iron deficiency. *Journal of the American Medical Association* 207: 552–53.

1997. Update: Blood lead levels—United States, 1991–1994. *MMWR: Morbidity and mortality weekly report* 46: 141–46.

2000. *Oxford English dictionary.* Oxford: Oxford UP.

2006 (Apr. 27). Mud pie keeps girl in good health. *China Daily* (*see* www.chinadaily .com.cn/china/2006–04/27/content_578036.htm). Accessed Dec. 5, 2006.

Aagaard-Hansen, J., and J. H. Ouma. 2002. Managing interdisciplinary health research: Theoretical and practical aspects. *International Journal of Health Planning and Management* 17: 195–212.

Abrahams, P., M. Follansbee, A. Hunt, B. Smith, and J. Wragg. 2006. Iron nutrition and possible lead toxicity: An appraisal of geophagy undertaken by pregnant women of UK Asian communities. *Applied Geochemistry* 21: 98–108.

Abu-Hamdan, D. K., J. H. Sondheimer, and S. K. Mahajan. 1985. Cautopyreiophagia: Cause of life-threatening hyperkalemia in a patient undergoing hemodialysis. *American Journal of Medicine* 79: 517–19.

Adam, I., A. H. Khamis, and M. I. Elbashir. 2005. Prevalence and risk factors for anaemia in pregnant women of eastern Sudan. *Transactions of the Royal Society of Tropical Medicine and Hygiene*: 739–43.

Aetius of Amida/J. V. Ricci. 1542 [1950]. *Aetios of Amida: The Gynaecology and Obstetrics of the Sixth Century*. Philadelphia: Blakiston.

Al-kanhal, M. A., and I. A. Bani. 1995. Food habits during pregnancy among Saudi women. *International Journal for Vitamin and Nutrition Research* 65: 206–10.

Allan, J. D., and J. Woodruff. 1963. Starch gastrolith: Report of a case of obstruction. *New England Journal of Medicine* 268: 776–78.

Amerson, J. R., and H. Q. Jones. 1967. Prolonged kaolin (clay) ingestion: A cause of colon perforation and peritonitis. *Bulletin of the Emory University Clinic* 5: 11–15.

Anderson, J., M. Akmal, and D. Kittur. 1991. Surgical complications of pica: Report of a case of intestinal obstruction and a review of the literature. *American Surgeon* 57: 663–67.

Anderson, O. 2005. Self-diagnosis: Your workouts can reveal what's wrong with your health (*see* www.pponline.co.uk/encyc/0201.htm). Accessed June 4, 2007.

Anell, B., and S. Lagercrantz. 1958. *Geophagical Customs*. Uppsala: Studia Ethnographica Upsaliensia.

Antelman, G., G. Msamanga, D. Spiegelman, E. Urassa, R. Narh, D. Hunter et al. 2000. Nutritional factors and infectious disease contribute to anemia among pregnant women with human immunodeficiency virus in Tanzania. *Journal of Nutrition* 130: 1950–57.

Anziulewicz, J. A., H. J. Dick, and E. E. Chiarulli. 1959. Transplacental naphthalene poisoning. *American Journal of Obstetrics and Gynecology* 78: 519–21.

Arcasoy, A., A. Cavdar, and E. Babacan. 1978. Decreased iron and zinc absorption in Turkish children with iron deficiency and geophagia. *Acta Haematologica* 60: 76–84.

Arenas, R. 2000. *Before night falls*. New York: Penguin Books.

Aristotle. 1897. *The Nichomachean Ethics of Aristotle*. London: MacMillan.

Armstrong, S. H., and R. F. Kourany. 1979. Iatrogenic deterioration and hemodialysis. *Journal of the Tennessee Medical Association* 72: 883–85.

Associated Press. 1988 (Dec 3). Eating dirt hard habit to break. *Toronto Star*, J2.

Associated Press. 1995 (June 2). Just spell him C-H-A-M-P: Arkansas 8th-grader wins National Bee. *Charleston Gazette* (W. Va.), 12A.

Aufreiter, S., W. Mahaney, M. W. Milner, M. Huffman, R. Hancock, M. Wink et al. 2001. Mineralogical and chemical interactions of soils eaten by chimpanzees of the Mahale Mountains and Gombe Stream National Parks, Tanzania. *Journal of Chemical Ecology* 27: 285–311.

Barlow, C. C. 2000. *The ghosts of evolution: Nonsensical fruit, missing partners, and other ecological anachronisms*. New York: Basic Books.

Barltrop, D. 1966. The prevalence of pica. *American Journal of Diseases of Children* 112: 116–23.

Basden, G. T. 1938. *Niger Ibos: A description of the primitive life, customs and animistic beliefs, &c., of the Ibo people of Nigeria by one who, for thirty-five years, enjoyed the privilege of their intimate confidence and friendship*. London: Seeley, Service.

Bear, I. J., and R. G. Thomas. 1964. Nature of argillaceous odour. *Nature* 201: 993–95.

Bearer, C. 1995. Environmental health hazards: How children are different from adults. *The Future of Children* 5: 11–26.

Beck, D, and N. Frohberg. 2005. Coprophagia in an elderly man: A case report and review of the literature. *International Journal of Psychiatry in Medicine* 35: 417–27.

Beecroft, N., L. Bach, N. Tunstall, and R. Howard. 1998. An unusual case of pica. *International Journal of Geriatric Psychiatry* 13: 638–41.

Belon, P. 1588. *Les observations de plvsievrs singvlaritez et choses memorables, trouvees en Grece, Asie, Indée, Egypte, Arabie, & autres pays étranges, redigées en trois livres*. Paris: H. de Marnef, & la veufue G. Cauellat.

Berg, J. M, and M. Zappella. 1964. Lead poisoning in childhood with particular reference to pica and mental sequelae. *Journal of Mental Deficiency Research* 42: 44–53.

Betten, H. F. 1687. *Disputatio medica inauguralis, de pica*. Trajecti ad Rhenum: Ex officina Francisci Halma.

Bhalla, J. N., P. K. Khanna, J. R. Srivastava, B. K. Sur, and M. Bhalla. 1983. Serum zinc level in pica. *Indian Pediatrics* 20: 667–70.

Biot, P. M. 1839. Note sur des matieres pierreuses employées a la Chine dans les temps de famine, sous le nom de Farine de Pierre. *Annales de Chimie et de Physique* 62: 215–19.

Black, D. A. K. 1956 (Oct. 27). A re-evaluation of terra sigilatta. *Lancet* 268.6948: 883–84.

Blount, R. 1988. *Now, where were we?* New York: Villard Books.

Blum, M., C. Orton, and L. Rose. 1968. The effect of starch ingestion on excessive iron absorption. *Annals of Internal Medicine* 68: 1165.

Bolton, K., V. M. Campbell, and F. D. Burton. 1998. Chemical analysis of soils of Kowloon (Hong Kong) eaten by hybrid macaques. *Journal of Chemical Ecology* 24: 195–205.

Bourke, J. G., B. Loewy, and E. W. Osborner. 1884. *The snake-dance of the Moquis of Arizona*. New York: Scribner's.

Bourne, J. K. 2008 (Sept.). Dirt Poor. *National Geographic*: 108–11.

Boyle, T. C. 1987. *World's end*. New York: Viking.

Bradley, F. W. 1964. Sandlappers and clay eaters. *North Carolina Folklore* 12: 27–28.

Bradley, J. E., and S. P. Bessman. 1958. Poverty, pica, and poisoning. *Public Health Reports* 73: 467–68.

Bridgens, R. Sketches of West India Scenery, with Illustrations of Negro Character, the Process of making Sugar, etc, from Sketches Taken during a Voyage to and a

Residence of Seven Years in the Island of Trinidad, 1836. London: Robert Jennings. (For fig. 6.2 of the present volume: Image Reference BRIDG-4_IMG, as shown on www.slaveryimages.org, sponsored by the Virginia Foundation for the Humanities and the University of Virginia Library). Accessed Dec. 12, 2009.

Brock, A. J. 1929. Greek medicine, being extracts illustrative of medical writers from Hippocrates to Galen. London: Dent.

Bronstein, E. S., and J. Dollar. 1974. Pica in pregnancy. *Journal of the Medical Association of Georgia* 63: 332–35.

Browman, D. L., and J. N. Gunderson. 1993. Altiplano comestible earths: Prehistoric and historic geophagy of highland Peru and Bolivia. *Geoarcheology* 8: 413–25.

Brown, D., and R. Juhl. 1976. Decreased bioavailability of digoxin due to antacids and kaolin-pectin. *New England Journal of Medicine* 295: 1034–37.

Brown, W., and P. Dyment. 1972. Pagophagia and iron deficiency anemia in adolescent girls. *Pediatrics* 49: 766–67.

Browne, P. 1756. *The civil and natural history of Jamaica: In three parts . . . In three dissertations. The whole illustrated with fifty copper-plates: in which the most curious productions are represented of the natural size, and delineated immediately from the objects.* London: Printed for the author, and sold to T. Osborne and J. Shipton, in Gray's-Inn.

Brugsch, H. K. 1886. *Im Lande der Sonne: Wanderungen in Persien.* Berlin: Allgemeiner Verein für Deutsche Literatur.

Brunhuber, K. B. 2008 (July 16). Doctors, activists work to stop clay eating in Africa. *Globe and Mail* (*see* www.theglobeandmail.com/servlet/story/RTGAM .20080716.wclay16/BNStory/International/home).

Buchanan, G. 1999. The tragedy of iron deficiency during infancy and early childhood. *Journal of Pediatrics* 135: 413–15.

Buck, P. H. 1925. The poor whites of the antebellum South. *American Historical Review* 31: 41–54.

Buck, P. S. 1994 [1931]. *The good earth.* New York: Pocket Book Classics.

Buckingham, J. S. 1842. *The slave states of America.* Vol. 1. London and Paris: Fisher.

Budge, E. A. W. 1913. *Syrian anatomy, pathology and therapeutics; or, "The Book of Medicines.* London: Oxford UP.

Burke, E. P. 1978 [1871]. *Pleasure and pain, reminiscences of Georgia in the 1840's.* Savannah: Beehive Press.

Buschan, G. 1930. Vom Erde-essen. *Janus* 34: 337–50.

Butler, P. M. 1982. Pica practices as an influence on iron deficiency anemia. MS thesis, East Carolina University, Greenville, N.C.

Calabrese, E. J., E. J. Stanek, R. C. James, and S. M. Roberts. 1999. Soil ingestion: A concern for acute toxicity in children. *Journal of Environmental Health* 61: 18–25.

Callahan, G. 2003. Eating dirt. *Emerging Infectious Diseases* 9: 1016–21.

Campbell, L., D. G. Dixon, and R. E. Hecky. 2003. A review of mercury in Lake Victoria, East Africa: Implications for human and ecosystem health. *Journal of Toxicology and Environmental Health, Part B* 6: 325–56.

Canaan, T. 1925. Mohammedan Saints and Sanctuaries in Palestine. *Journal of the Palestine Oriental Society* 5: 163–203.

Carlander, O. 1959. Aetiology of pica. *Lancet* 2: 569.

Carpenter, W. M. 1844. Observations on the Cachexia Africana, or the habit and effects of dirt-eating in the negro race. *New Orleans Medical Journal* 1: 146–68.

Cavdar, A., and A. Arcasoy. 1972. Hematologic and biochemical studies of Turkish children with pica: A presumptive explanation for the syndrome of geophagia, iron deficiency anemia, hepatosplenomegaly, and hypogonadism. *Clinical Pediatrics* 11: 215–23.

Cavdar, A. O., A. Arcasoy, S. Cin, E. Babacan, and S. Gozdasoglu. 1983. Geophagia in Turkey: Iron and zinc absorption studies and response to treatment with zinc in geophagia cases. In A. Prasad, A. O. Cavdar, G. Brewer, and P. Aggett, eds., *Zinc deficiency in human subjects: Proceedings of an international symposium held in Ankara, Turkey, April 29–30, 1982,* 71–97. New York: A. R. Liss.

Cavdar, A. O., A. Arcasoy, S. Cin, and H. Gumus. 1980. Zinc deficiency in geophagia in Turkish children and response to treatment with zinc sulphate. *Haematologica* 65: 403–408.

Celsus, A. C./Grieve, J. 1756. *Of Medicine.* Cambridge: Harvard UP.

Cervantes/Grossman, E., and H. Bloom. 2003. *Don Quixote* (Pt. 1, 1605; pt. 2, 1615). New York: Ecco.

Chen, X, T. Yin, J. He, Q. Ma, Z. Han, and L. Li. 1985. Low levels of zinc in hair and blood, pica, anorexia, and poor growth in Chinese preschool children. *American Journal of Clinical Nutrition* 42: 694–700.

Chisholm, C. 1799. Account of the Cachexia Africana; a Disease incidental to Negro Slaves lately imported into the West-Indies. *Medical Repository of Original Essays and Intelligence*: 282–84.

Chisholm, J. C., and H. I. Martin. 1981. Hypozincemia, ageusia, dysosmia, and toilet tissue pica. *Journal of the National Medical Association* 73: 163–64.

Chopra, R. N. 1933. *Indigenous drugs of India: Their medical and economic aspects.* Calcutta: The Art Press.

Christiani, D. 1691. *Dissertatio medica de pica.* Francofurti ad Viadrum: Literis Christophori Zeitleri.

Clark, J. D. 2001. *Kalambo Falls prehistoric site.* Vol. 3. London: Cambridge UP.

Cleaton, S. 1983 (June 11). Queens doctor wages long fight to stop black women from eating starch. *New York Voice.*

Cobo, B., and J. M. de la Espada. 1890. *Historia del Nuevo mundo.* Sevilla: Imp. de E. Rasco.

Cohen, G. J., R. S. Lourie, and W. Abernethy. 1965. Grand rounds: Pica and lead poisoning. *Clinical Proceedings of the Children's Hospital of District of Columbia* 21: 193–204.

Cole, F., and A. Gale. 1922. *The Tinguian: Social, religious, and economic life of a Philippine tribe*. Chicago: Field Museum of Natural History.

Coles, T., J. Schall, M. Hediger, and T. Scholl. 1995. Pica during pregnancy—associations with dietary intake, serum micronutrients and pregnancy outcome. *FASEB Journal* 9: A443.

Coltman, C. J. 1969. Pagophagia and iron lack. *Journal of the American Medical Association* 207: 513–16.

Coltman, C. J. 1971. Pagophagia. *Archives of Internal Medicine* 128: 472–73.

Conrad, M. K. 1979. An examination of the environmental and psychological correlates of lead poisoning in young children. Ph.D. diss., University of Wisconsin, Milwaukee.

Cooksey, N. 1995. Pica and olfactory craving of pregnancy: How deep are the secrets? *Birth* 22: 129–37.

Cooney, D. O. 1995. *Activated charcoal in medical applications*. New York: Dekker.

Cooney, D. O., and T. T. Struhsaker. 1997. Adsorptive capacity of charcoals eaten by Zanzibar red colobus monkeys: Implications for reducing dietary toxins. *International Journal of Primatology* 18: 235–46.

Cooper, M. M. 1957. *Pica: A survey of the historical literature as well as reports from the fields of veterinary medicine and anthropology, the present study of pica in young children, and a discussion of its pediatric and psychological implications*. Springfield, Ill: Thomas.

Corbett, R., C. Ryan, and S. Weinrich. 2003. Pica in pregnancy: Does it affect pregnancy outcomes? *American Journal of Maternal and Child Nursing* 28: 183–89; quiz, 90–91.

Costermans. 1895. Le District du Stanley-Pool. *Bulletin de la Société d'Études Coloniales* 2: 25–52.

Cotting, J. R. 1836. Analysis of a species of clay found in Richmond County which is eagerly sought after and eaten by many people, particularly children. *Southern Medical and Surgical Journal* 1: 288–92.

Coulombe M. 2007. Arizona State University. Healing clays (*see* http://researchstories.asu.edu/stories/healing-clay-906). Accessed Dec. 20, 2009.

Courbon, B., J. Boulloche, and E. Mallet. 1987. [Plaster geophagia in an immigrant Maugrabin child]. *Archives français de pédiatrie* 44: 145.

Courlander, H. 1976. *A treasury of Afro-American folklore: The oral literature, traditions, recollections, legends, tales, songs, religious beliefs, customs, sayings, and humor of peoples of African descent in the Americas*. New York: Crown.

Cragin, F. W. 1835. Observations on Cachexia Africana or Dirt-Eating. *American Journal of the Medical Sciences* 17: 356–64.

Crosby, W. H. 1976a. Pica. *Journal of the American Medical Association* 235: 2765.

Crosby, W. H. 1976b. Pica: A compulsion caused by iron deficiency. *British Journal of Haematology* 34: 341–42.

Dahms, P. 1897. Uber Bergmehl und Diatomeenführende Schichten in Westpreussen. *Naturwissenschaftliche Wochenschrift* 12: 385–88.

Danford, D., J. J. Smith, A. Huber. 1982. Pica and mineral status in the mentally retarded. *American Journal of Clinical Nutrition* 35: 958–67.

Dannenfeldt, K. 1984. The introduction of a new sixteenth-century drug: Terra Silesiaca. *Medical History* 28: 174–88.

Davenport, G. 1980. The anthropology of table manners from geophagy onward. *Antaeus* 36: 136–43.

Day, S. 2000 (Oct. 29). Jamaica Journal: An old-fashioned country doctor finishes his last rounds in the big city. *New York Times* (*see* www.nytimes.com/2000/10/29/nyregion/jamaica-journal-old-fashioned-country-doctor-finishes-his-last-rounds-big-city.html?pagewanted=1).

De Borhegyi, S. F. 1954. The cult of Our Lord of Esquipulas in Middle America and New Mexico. *El Palacio* 61: 387–401.

De Castro, J., and J. Boyd-Orr. 1952. *The geography of hunger*. Boston: Little Brown.

De Hoyos Sáinz, L., and N. de Hoyos Sancho. 1947. *Manual de folklore, la vida popular tradicional*. Madrid: Revista de Occidente.

De la Burde, B., and B. Reames. 1973. Prevention of pica, the major cause of lead poisoning in children. *American Journal of Public Health* 63: 737–43.

De Torquemada, J. 1723. *Monarquía indiana*. Madrid: N. Rodriquez Franco.

Dean, J. R., M. E. Deary, B. K. Gbefa, and W. C. Scott. 2004. Characterisation and analysis of persistent organic pollutants and major, minor and trace elements in Calabash chalk. *Chemosphere* 57: 21–25.

Debret, J. B. 1835. Voyage pittoresque et historique au Brésil, ou Séjour d'un artiste français au Brésil, depuis 1816 jusqu'en 1831 inclusivement, epoque de l'avénement et de l'abdication de S. M. D. Pedro 1er, fondateur de l'Empire brésilien. Rio de Janeiro, New York: Distribuidora Record, Continental News.

Den Hollander, A. N. J. 1935. The tradition of "poor whites." In W. Cough, ed., *Culture in the South*, 403–31. Chapel Hill: U of North Carolina P.

Diamond, J., K. D. Bishop, and J. D. Gilardi. 1999. Geophagy in New Guinea birds. *Ibis* 141: 181–93.

Díaz del Castillo, B., G. García, A. P. Maudslay, and M. H. Saville. 1908. *The true history of the conquest of New Spain*. London: Printed for the Hakluyt Society.

Dickins, D., and R. N. Ford. 1942. Geophagy (dirt-eating) among Mississippi Negro schoolchildren. *American Sociological Review* 7: 59–65.

Dioscorides, P./Goodyer, J. and R. T. Gunther. 1934. *The Greek Herbal of Dioscorides*. Oxford: Printed by J. Johnson for the author.

Diouf, S., B. Camara, M. G. Sall, I. Diagne, O. Ndiaye, A. Diallo et al. 2000. [Protein-energy malnutrition in children less than five years old in a rural zone in Senegal (Khombole)]. *Dakar médical* 45: 48–50.

Dominy, N., E. Davoust, and M. Minekus. 2004. Adaptive function of soil consumption: An in vitro study modeling the human stomach and small intestine. *Journal of Experimental Biology* 207: 319–24.

Dors [Dons], J. L. 1838. Récherches sur la Cachexie Africaine. *Gazette médicale de Paris* 6: 289–95.

Dreyer, M. J., P. G. Chaushev, and R. F. Gledhill. 2004. Biochemical investigations in geophagia. *Journal of the Royal Society of Medicine* 97: 48.

Du Halde, J. 1741. *The general history of China: Containing a geographical, historical, chronological, political and physical description of the Empire of China adorn'd with curious maps, and copper plates.* London: Printed by and for J. Watts at the Printing-Office near Wild-Courts near Lincolns-Inn Fields.

Dunston, B. N. 1961. Pica, hemoglobin, and prematurity and perinatal mortality: An experimental investigation of the relationships between pica, hemoglobin levels, and prematurity and perinatal mortality among a clinic population of married Negro pregnant women. Doctor of Education diss. New York University, New York.

Duprey, A. J. B. 1900. The anaemia of dyspepsia consequent on dirt-eating. *Lancet* 2: 1192–93.

Dutt, U. C., B. L. Sen, A. Sen, and P. K. Sen. 1980. *The materia medica of the Hindus.* Varanasi: Chowkhamba Saraswatibhawan.

Ebers, G. 1889. *Papyrus Ebers: Die Maasse und das Kapitel über die Augenkrankheiten.* Leipzig: S. Hirzel.

Eckholm, E. 1986 (July 1). Clay eating proves widespread but reason is uncertain. *New York Times.*

Edwards, C., A. Johnson, E. Knight, U. Oyemade, O. Cole, O. Westney et al. 1994. Pica in an urban environment. *Journal of Nutrition* 124: 954S–962S.

Edwards, C. H., S. Mcdonald, J. R. Mitchell, and L. Jones. 1964. Effect of clay and cornstarch intake on women and their infants. *Journal of the American Dietetic Association* 44: 109–15.

Edwards, C. H., S. McDonald, J. R. Mitchell, L. Jones, L. Mason, A. M. Kemp et al. 1959. Clay- and cornstarch-eating women. *Journal of the American Dietetic Association* 35: 810–15.

Edwards, C. H., H. McSwain, and S. Haire. 1954. Odd dietary practices of women. *Journal of the American Dietetic Association* 30: 976–81.

Ellis, R. P., M. P. Cochrane, and M. F. B. Dale. 1998. Starch production and industrial use. *Journal of the Science of Food and Agriculture* 77: 289–311.

Ellis, W. 1853. *Polynesian researches during a residence of nearly eight years in the Society and Sandwich Islands.* London: H. G. Bohn.

Farag, T., R. Stoltzfus, S. Khalfan, and J. Tielsch. 2007. Helicobacter pylori infection is associated with severe anemia of pregnancy on Pemba Island, Zanzibar. *American Journal of Tropical Medicine & Hygiene* 76: 541–48.

Ferguson, J. H., and A. G. Keaton. 1950. Studies of the diets of pregnant women in Mississippi: I. The ingestion of clay and laundry starch. *New Orleans Medical and Surgical Journal* 102: 460–63.

Ferrand, E. 1886. Terres comestibles de Java. *Revue d'Ethnographie* 5: 548–49.

Ferrell, R. E. 2008. Medicinal clay and spiritual healing. *Clays and Clay Minerals* 56: 751–60.

Fessler, D. 2002. Reproductive immunosuppression and diet. *Current Anthropology* 43: 19–60.

Finger, M. 1993 (Dec.). The clay eaters of Memphis. *Memphis*: 11.

Firth, D. 2004. *Salad Fingers* (see www.fat-pie.com/salad.htm). Accessed Mar. 28, 2009.

Fisher, J. R., M. L. Sievers, R. T. Takeshita, and H. Caldwell. 1981. Skeletal fluorosis from eating soil. *Arizona Medicine* 38: 833–35.

Flaxman, S., and P. Sherman. 2000. Morning sickness: A mechanism for protecting mother and embryo. *Quarterly Review of Biology* 75: 113–48.

Forestus, P./Burri, R. 1982 [1557]. *Die Delfter Pest von 1557 nach den Beobachtungen von Petrus Forestus*. Zürich: Juris Druck + Verlag.

Forsyth, C., and G. M. Benoit. 1989. "Rare, Old, Dirty Snacks": Some research notes on dirt eating. *Deviant Behavior* 10: 61–68.

Fossey, D. 1983. *Gorillas in the mist*. Boston: Houghton Mifflin.

Foster, J. W. 1927. Pica. *Kenya and East African Medical Journal*: 68–76.

François, B., and O. Brenet. 2004. Medical mystery—the answer. *New England Journal of Medicine* 350: 839.

Frate, D. 1984. Last of the earth eaters. *The Sciences* 24: 34–38.

Furuseth, O. J. 1973. Geophagy in eastern North Carolina. MA thesis, East Carolina University, Greenville.

Galt, F. 1872. Medical notes on the upper Amazon. *American Journal of Medical Sciences* 128: 395–417.

García Márquez, G. 1998 [1967]. *One hundred years of solitude*. New York: Perennial Classics.

Garg, M., M. J. Shaver, and A. Easom. 2004. Pica: An underappreciated cause of electrolyte abnormalities. *Nephrology News and Issues* 18: 28–29, 33.

Garnier, J. 1871. *Voyage autour du monde: La nouvelle-calédonie (côte orientale)*. Paris: H. Plon.

Gautier, T., and T. R. McQuoid. 1853. *Wanderings in Spain*. London: Ingram, Cooke.

Geissler, P. W. 2000. The significance of earth-eating: Social and cultural aspects of geophagy among Luo children. *Africa* 70: 653–82.

Geissler, P., D. Mwaniki, F. Thiong'o, and H. Friis. 1997. Geophagy among school children in western Kenya. *Tropical Medicine and International Health* 2: 624–30.

Geissler, P., D. Mwaniki, F. Thiong'o, and H. Friis. 1998a. Geophagy as a risk factor for geohelminth infections: A longitudinal study of Kenyan primary schoolchildren. *Transactions of the Royal Society of Tropical Medicine and Hygiene* 92: 7–11.

Geissler, P., C. Shulman, R. Prince, W. Mutemi, C. Mnazi, H. Friis et al. 1998b. Geophagy, iron status and anaemia among pregnant women on the coast of Kenya. *Transactions of the Royal Society of Tropical Medicine and Hygiene* 92: 549–53.

Gelfand, M. 1945. Geophagy and its relation to hookworm disease. *East African Medical Journal* 22: 98–103.

Gelfand, M., A. Zarate, and J. H. Knepshield. 1975. Geophagia: A cause of life-threatening hyperkalemia in patients with chronic renal failure. *Journal of the American Medical Association* 234: 738–40.

Georgette, K., and T. Francis. 2003. A study of the hydrochloric acid (HCl) extractable mineral components of a clay substance eaten in Ghana. University of Ghana, Department of Nutrition and Food Sciences: unpublished manuscript.

Gerber, N. N., and H. A. Lechevalier. 1965. Geosmin, an earthly-smelling substance isolated from actinomycetes. *Applied Microbiology* 13: 935–38.

Gibbons, K. 1988. *Ellen Foster*. New York: Vintage Books.

Gilardi, J. D., S. S. Duffey, C. A. Munn, and L. A. Tell. 1999. Biochemical functions of geophagy in parrots: Detoxification of dietary toxins and cytoprotective effects. *Journal of Chemical Ecology* 25: 897–922.

Gilmore, J. R. 1862. *Among the pines or, South in secession-time*. New York: Charles T. Evans.

Giudicelli, J., and J. C. Combes. 1992. [Pica and iron deficiency in adolescence]. *Archives français de pédiatrie* 49: 779–83.

Gladfelter, J., B. Einspruch, and B. Black. 1960. The study of pica and food preferences in a postpartum general hospital population. *Texas Reports on Biology and Medicine* 18: 202–204.

Glickman, L., I. Chaudry, J. Costantino, F. Clack, R. Cypess, and L. Winslow. 1981. Pica patterns, toxocariasis, and elevated blood lead in children. *American Journal of Tropical Medicine & Hygiene* 30: 77–80.

Gomme, L. G. 1892. *Ethnology in folklore*. London: Kegan, Paul, Trench, Trubner.

Gonzalez, J. J., W. Owens, P. C. Ungaro, E. E. Werk, and P. W. Wentz. 1982. Clay ingestion: A rare cause of hypokalemia. *Annals of Internal Medicine* 97: 65–66.

Gonzalez, R., F. S. De Medina, O. Martinez-Augustin, A. Nieto, J. Galvez, S. Risco et al. 2004. Anti-inflammatory effect of diosmectite in hapten-induced colitis in the rat. *British Journal of Pharmacology* 141: 951–60.

Good, B., C. V. Holland, M. R. Taylor, J. Larragy, P. Moriarty, and M. O'Regan. 2004. Ocular toxocariasis in schoolchildren. *Clinical Infectious Diseases* 39: 173–78.

Goodman, A. H., and T. L. Leatherman. 1998. *Building a new biocultural synthesis: Political-economic perspectives on human biology*. Ann Arbor: U of Michigan P.

Graham, P. W. 1976. Stercoraceous perforation of the pelvic colon—an unusual complication of pica. *Medical Journal of Australia* 2: 385–86.

Green, H. H. 1925. Perverted appetites. *Physiological Review* 5: 336–48.

Green, M. H. 2001. *Trotula Major: A medieval compendium of women's medicine*. Philadelphia: U of Pennsylvania P.

Greenberg, L. W. 1977. Pica and parotitis. *Hospital Practice* 12: 25.

Gregory, P. 2007. *A respectable trade*. New York: Simon and Schuster.

Grigsby, R., B. Thyer, R. Waller, and G. J. Johnston. 1999. Chalk eating in middle Georgia: A culture-bound syndrome of pica? *Southern Medical Journal* 92: 190–92.

Guernier, V., M. Hochberg, and J. Guegan. 2004. Ecology drives the worldwide distribution of human diseases. *PLoS Biology* 2: e141.

Guiges, P. 1905. Les noms arabes dans Sérapion. *Journal Asiatique* 5: 85.

Gutelius, M. F., F. K. Millican, E. M. Layman, G. J. Cohen, and C. C. Dublin. 1962. Nutritional studies of children with pica I. Controlled study evaluating nutritional status II. Treatment of pica with iron given intramuscularly. *Pediatrics* 29: 1018–23.

Gutelius, M. F., F. K. Millican, E. M. Layman, G. J. Cohen, and C. C. Dublin. 1963. Treatment of pica with a vitamin and mineral supplement. *American Journal of Clinical Nutrition* 12: 388–93.

Haanen, H. C., and H. L. Tan-tjiong. 1982. [A patient with pagophagia and iron deficiency anemia]. *Nederlands Tijdschrift voor Geneeskunde* 126: 2379–80.

Haberlandt, M. 1899. Contraire Sexual-Erscheinungen bei der Neger-Bevolkerung Zanzibars. *Zeitschrift fur Ethnologie* 31: 668–70.

Hall, A., and E. Photos-Jones. 2008. Accessing past beliefs and practices: The case of Lemnian earth. *Archaeometry* 50: 1034–49.

Halsted, J. 1968. Geophagia in man: Its nature and nutritional effects. *American Journal of Clinical Nutrition* 21: 1384–93.

Hamilton, S., S. J. Rothenberg, F. A. Khan, M. Manalo, and K. C. Norris. 2001. Neonatal lead poisoning from maternal pica behavior during pregnancy. *Journal of the National Medical Association* 93: 317–19.

Hamy, E. T. 1899. Les géophages du Tonkin. *Bulletin du Museum d'historie naturelle* 5: 64–66.

Hancock, J. 1831. Remarks on the common cachexia or leucophlegmasia called mal d'estomac in the colonies and its kindred affections, as dropsy, etc. *Edinburgh Medical and Surgical Journal* 35: 67–73.

Handler, J., and A. Steiner. 2006. Identifying pictorial images of Atlantic slavery: Three case studies. *Slavery and Abolition* 27: 51–71.

Harper, B. L., B. Flett, S. Harris, C. Abeyta, and F. Kirschner. 2002. The Spokane Tribe's multipathway subsistence exposure scenario and screening level RME. *Risk Analysis* 22: 513–26.

Harries, J., and T. Hughes. 1958 (July). Enumerations of the "cravings" of some pregnant women. *British Medical Journal* 5: 39–40.

Hasan, N., D. Emery, S. Baithun, and S. Dodd. 1995. Chronic copper intoxication due to ingestion of coins: A report of an unusual case. *Human and Experimental Toxicology* 14: 500–502.

Hasluck, F. 1909. Terra Lemnia. *Annual of the British School at Athens* 16: 220–23.

Hassan, H. A., C. Netchvolodoff, and J. P. Raufman. 2000. Zinc-induced copper deficiency in a coin swallower. *American Journal of Gastroenterology* 95: 2975–77.

Hawkesworth, John. 1773. *An account of the voyages undertaken by the order of His Present Majesty for making discoveries in the Southern Hemisphere and successively perfored by Commodore Byron, Captain Wallis, Captain Carteret, and Captain Cook, in the Dolphin, the Swallow, and the Endeavor.* Vol. 2. London: Printed for W. Strahan; and T. Cadell in the Strand.

Haydel, S. E., C. M. Remenih, and L. B. Williams. 2008. Broad-spectrum in vitro antibacterial activities of clay minerals against antibiotic-susceptible and antibiotic-resistant bacterial pathogens. *Journal of Antimicrobial Chemotherapy* 61: 353–61.

Henon, P., I. Gerota, and J. Caen. 1975. [Letter: One can remain a geophagist in Paris]. *La Nouvelle Presse Médicale* 4: 1431.

Henry, J., and A. M. Kwong. 2003. Why is geophagy treated like dirt? *Deviant Behavior* 24: 353–71.

Hertz, H. 1947. Notes on clay and starch eating among Negroes in a Southern urban community. *Social Forces* 25: 343–44.

Hewson, A. 1872. *Earth as a topical application in surgery: Being a full exposition of its use in all the cases requiring topical applications admitted in the men's and women's surgical wards of the Pennsylvania Hospital during a period of six months in 1869.* Philadelphia: Lindsay and Blakiston.

Hippocrates. 1853. *Oeuvres Complètes d'Hippocrate.* Vol. 8. Paris: J. B. Baillière.

Hladik, C. M., and L. Gueguen. 1974. Geophagie et nutrition minerale chez les primates sauvages. *Comptes rendus de l'Academie des sciences Serie III* 279: 1393–96.

Holt, A., R. Spargo, J. Iveson, G. Faulkner, and D. Cheek. 1980. Serum and plasma zinc, copper and iron concentrations in Aboriginal communities of North Western Australia. *American Journal of Clinical Nutrition* 33: 119–32.

Holt, W., and C. Hendricks. 1969. Dysfunctional labor due to fecal impaction: Report of a case. *Obstetrics and Gynecology* 34: 502–505.

Hooda, P. S., C. J. Henry, T. A. Seyoum, L. D. Armstrong, and M. B. Fowler MB. 2004. The potential impact of soil ingestion on human mineral nutrition. *Science of the Total Environment* 333: 75–87.

Hooper, D., and H. H. Mann. 1906. Earth-eating and the earth-eating habit in India. *Memoirs of the Asiatic Society of Bengal* 1: 249–73.

Hopffe, A. 1917. Uber infusorienerde (Bergmehl). *Naturwissenschaftliche Wochenschrift* 16: 286–87.

Houston, D., J. Gilardi, and J. Hall. 2001. Soil consumption by elephants might help to minimize the toxic effects of plant secondary compounds in forest browse. *Mammal Review* 31: 249–54.

Howarth. S., and E. R. Lamadrid. 1999. *Pilgrimage to Chimayó: Contemporary portrait of a living tradition.* Santa Fe: Museum of New Mexico Press.

Hudson, R. P. 1977. The biography of disease: Lessons from chlorosis. *Bulletin of the History of Medicine* 51: 448–63.

Hui, C. A. 2004. Geophagy and potential contaminant exposure for terrestrial vertebrates. *Reviews of Environmental Contamination & Toxicology* 183: 115–34.

Hui, Y., R. Smith, and D. Spoerke. 2001a. *Foodborne Disease Handbook*, vol. 1: *Diseases Caused by Bacteria*. New York: Marcel Dekker.

Hui, Y., R. Smith, and D. Spoerke. 2001b. *Foodborne Disease Handbook*, vol. 3: *Plant Toxicants*. New York: Marcel Dekker.

Hunter, J. 1788. *Observations on the diseases of the army in Jamaica; and on the best means of preserving the health of Europeans, in that climate*. London: Printed for G. Nicol.

Hunter, J. 1984. Insect clay geophagy in Sierra Leone. *Journal of Cultural Geography* 4: 2–13.

Hunter, J. M. 1973. Geophagy in Africa and in the United States: A culture-nutrition hypothesis. *Geographical Review* 63: 170–95.

Hunter, J. M. 1993. Macroterme geophagy and pregnancy clays in southern Africa. *Journal of Cultural Geography* 14: 69–92.

Hunter, J. M., and R. de Kleine. 1984. Geophagy in Central America. *Geographical Review* 74: 157–69.

Hunter, J. M., O. H. Horst, and R. N. Thomas. 1989. Religious geophagy as a cottage industry: The holy clay tablet of Esquipulas, Guatemala. *National Geographic Research* 5: 281–95.

Hurston, Z. N. 1935. *Of Mules and Men*. Philadelphia and London: Lippincott.

Hussey, H. H. 1975 (editorial). Geophagia-induced hyperkalemia. *Journal of the American Medical Association* 234: 746.

Hyatt, H. M. 1970. *Hoodoo—conjuration—witchcraft—rootwork; beliefs accepted by many Negroes and White persons, these being orally recorded among Blacks and Whites*. Hannibal, Mo.: Printed by Western Pub., distributed by American University Bookstore.

Hyslop, N. S. G. 1977. Pica in man and animals. *British Journal of Haematology* 37: 154–55.

Ibn el-Beithar, and L. Leclerc. 1877. *Traité des simples (Djami el-Moufridat)*. Paris: Imprimerie Nationale.

Imray, J. 1843. Observations on the mal d'estomac or cachexia Africana, as it takes place among the Negroes of Dominica. *Edinburgh Medical and Surgical Journal* 59: 304–21.

Institute of Medicine. 1992. *Nutrition during pregnancy and lactation: An implementation guide*. Washington, D.C.: National Academy Press.

Institute of Medicine. 2002. DRI: Dietary Reference Intakes for vitamin A, vitamin K, arsenic, boron, chromium, copper, iodine, iron, manganese, molybdenum, nickel, silicon, vanadium, and zinc. Washington, D.C.: National Academy Press.

Jameson, S. 1971. [Bone marrow iron deposits—iron deficiency symptoms among 84 first pregnancies—a longitudinal study]. *Nordisk Medicin* 86: 1290.

Jee, H. H. B. S. 1896. *A short history of Aryan medical science.* London: Macmillan.

Jellingshaus, K. 1877. Ausflug von Jerusalem nach dem Todten Meere. *Mittheilungen des Vereins für Erdkunde zu Halle:* 47–67.

Jerome, N. W., R. F. Kandel, and G. H. Pelto. 1980. An ecological approach to nutritional anthropology. In N. W. Jerome, R. F. Kandel, and G. H. Pelto, eds., *Nutritional Anthropology: Contemporary Approaches to Diet and Culture,* 13–45. New York: Redgrave.

Johns, T. 1986. Detoxification function of geophagy and domestication of the potato. *Journal of Chemical Ecology* 12: 635–46.

Johns, T. 1996. *The origins of human diet and medicine.* Tucson: U of Arizona P.

Johns, T., and M. Duquette. 1991a. Detoxification and mineral supplementation as functions of geophagy. *American Journal of Clinical Nutrition* 53: 448–56.

Johns, T., and M. Duquette. 1991b. Traditional detoxification of acorn bread with clay. *Ecology of Food and Nutrition* 25: 221–28.

Johnson, B., and R. Stephens. 1982. Geomelophagia: An unusual pica in iron-deficiency anemia. *American Journal of Medicine* 73: 931–32.

Johnston, H. H. 1897. British Central Africa: An attempt to give some account of a portion of the territories under British influence north of the Zambesi. London: Methuen.

Kalayci, A., Y. Kanber, A. Birinci, L. Yildiz, and D. Albayrak. 2005. The prevalence of coeliac disease as detected by screening in children with iron deficiency anaemia. *Acta Paediatrica* 94: 678–81.

Kale, M. R. 1997. *The Raghuvamsha of Kalidasa, with the commentary of Sanjivani of Mallinatha, Cantos I-V.* Delhi: Motilal Banarsidass.

Karimi, M., R. Kadivar, and H. Yarmohammadi. 2002. Assessment of the prevalence of iron deficiency anemia, by serum ferritin, in pregnant women of Southern Iran. *Medical Science Monitor* 8: CR488–92.

Katz, J. 2008. National Geographic News. Poor Haitians resort to eating dirt (*see* http://news.nationalgeographic.com/news/2008/01/080130-AP-haiti-eatin.html). Accessed Apr. 18, 2008.

Katz, S. H., M. L. Hediger, and L. A. Valleroy. 1975. Traditional maize processing techniques in the New World. *Science* 184: 765–73.

Kawai, K., E. Saathoff, G. Antelman, G. Msamanga, W. W. Fawzi. 2009. Geophagy (Soil-eating) in relation to anemia and helminth infection among HIV-infected pregnant women in Tanzania. *American Journal of Tropical Medicine & Hygiene* 80: 36–43.

Keith, D., L. Keith, G. S. Berger, J. Foot, and A. Webster. 1975. Amylophagia during pregnancy: Some maternal and perinatal correlations. *Mount Sinai Journal of Medicine* 42: 410–14.

Keith, L., H. Evenhouse, and A. Webster. 1968. Amylophagia during pregnancy. *Obstetrics and Gynecology* 32: 415–18.

Kelsey, V, and L. Osborne. 1939. *Four keys to Guatemala.* New York and London: Funk and Wagnalls.

Kendall, N. R., and S. B. Telfer. 2000. Induction of zinc deficiency in sheep and its correction with a soluble glass bolus containing zinc. *Veterinary Record* 146: 634–37.

Kettaneh, A., V. Eclache, O. Fain, C. Sontag, M. Uzan, L. Carbillon et al. 2005. Pica and food craving in patients with iron-deficiency anemia: A case-control study in France. *American Journal of Medicine* 118: 185–88.

Key, T. J., E. Horger, and J. J. Miller. 1982. Geophagia as a cause of maternal death. *Obstetrics and Gynecology* 60: 525–26.

Khalil, S. A., N. A. Daabis, V. F. Naggar, and M. M. Motawi. 1976. The in vitro adsorption of some antibiotics on antacids. *Pharmazie* 31: 105–109.

Khanum, M. P. U. 1976. A survey of food habits and beliefs of pregnant and lactating mothers in Mysore city. *Indian Journal of Nutrition and Dietetics* 12: 208–17.

Kikouama, J. R., F. L. Cornec, S. Bouttier, A. Launay, L. Balde, and N. Yagoubi. 2008. Evaluation of trace elements released by edible clays in physicochemically simulated physiological media. *International Journal of Food Sciences and Nutrition* 60: 130–42.

Kingsolver, B. 1998. *The Poisonwood Bible*. London: Faber and Faber.

Kinietz, W. V., and A. D. Raudot. 1965. *The Indians of the western Great Lakes, 1615–1760*. Ann Arbor: U of Michigan P.

Kipling, R. 1893. One view of the question. In *Many inventions*, 79–105. New York: Appleton.

Kirsch, H. E. 1990. "Why do I crave that stuff?": Determinants of pica during pregnancy. BA thesis, Harvard University, Cambridge.

Klaus, G., and B. Schmid. 1998. Geophagy at natural licks and mammal ecology: A review. *Mammalia* 62: 481–97.

Klitzman, S., A. Sharma, L. Nicaj, R. Vitkevich, and J. Leighton. 2002. Lead poisoning among pregnant women in New York City: Risk factors and screening practices. *Journal of Urban Health* 79: 225–37.

Knishinsky, R. 1998. *The clay cure: Natural healing from the earth*. Rochester, Vt.: Healing Arts Press.

Korman, S. 1990. Pica as a presenting symptom in childhood celiac disease. *American Journal of Clinical Nutrition* 51: 139–41.

Kraemer, S. 2002. Clay, Vicks, and Gold Medal flour. *Southern Medical Journal* 95(10): 1228–29.

Kreulen, D. A. 1985. Lick use by large herbivores: A review of benefits and banes of soil consumption. *Mammalian Review* 15: 107–23.

Krishnamani, R., and W. Mahaney. 2000. Geophagy among primates: Adaptive significance and ecological consequences. *Animal Behavior* 59: 899–915.

Külz, L. 1919. Die Abhangigkeit der geistigen und kulturellen Ruckstandigkeit der Naturvolker von ihren endemischen Krankheiten. *Anthropos* 14: 33–45.

La Billardière, M. 1800. *An account of a voyage in search of la Pérouse, undertaken by ordor of the constituent assembly of France and performed in the years 1791,*

1792, 1793, *in the Recherche and Espérance, Ships of War*. Vol. 2. London: Printed for J. Debrett, Piccadilly.

Lamadrid, E. Mar. 1, 2001. On the road to Chimayo. *US Catholic*: 30–34.

Landman, J. P., and J. S. Hall. 1989. Dietary patterns and nutrition in pregnancy in Jamaica. *Journal of Tropical Pediatrics* 35: 185–90.

Landman, J. P., and J. S. Hall. 1992. Dietary habits and knowledge of folklore of pregnant Jamaican women. *Ecology of Food and Nutrition* 12: 203–10.

Lanzkowsky, P. 1959. Investigation into the aetiology and treatment of pica. *Archives of Disease in Childhood* 34: 140–48.

Laufer, B. 1930. *Geophagy*. Anthropological Series, vol. 18, no. 2 (monograph). Chicago: Field Museum of Natural History.

Lawson, J. 1967 [1709]. *A new voyage to Carolina*. Chapel Hill: U of North Carolina P.

Legey, F. 1926. *Essai de folklore Marocain*. Paris: Libraire Orientaliste Paul Geuthner.

Levacher, M. G. 1840. *Guide médical des Antilles*. Paris: Librairie médicale de Just Rouvier, Bureau du journal l'Outre-mer.

Libnoch, J. 1984. Geomelophagia: An unusual pica in iron-deficiency anemia. *American Journal of Medicine* 76: A69.

Liebault J. 1598. *Trois livres appartenans aux infirmitez et maladies des femmes*. Paris and Lyon: Veyrat.

Lithgow, W. 1632. *The totall discourse of the rare adventures & painefull peregrinations of long nineteene yeares travayles from Scotland to the most famous kingdomes in Europe, Asia and Affrica*. London: By Nicholas Okes, and are to be sold by Nicholas Fussell and Humphery Mosley at their shops in Pauls Church yard, at the Ball, and the white Lyon, 1632.

Liu, Y., N. Malik, G. Sanger, M. Friedman, and P. Andrews. 2005. Pica—a model of nausea? Species differences in response to cisplatin. *Physiology and Behavior* 85: 271–77.

Livingstone, D., and H. Waller. 1875. *The last journals of David Livingstone, in Central Africa, from eighteen hundred and sixty-five to his death*. New York: Harper and Brothers.

Lockwood Y. 1983. *Text and Context Folk-song in a Bosnian Muslim Village*. Columbus, Ohio: Slavica.

Lofts, R., S. Schroeder, and R. Maier. 1990. Effects of serum zinc supplementation on pica behavior of persons with mental retardation. *American Journal of Mental Retardation* 95: 103–109.

Logan, W. B. 1995. *Dirt: The ecstatic skin of the earth*. New York: Riverhead Books.

Longstreet, A. B. 1835. *Georgia scenes, characters, incidents, &c., in the first half century of the republic*. Augusta: Printed at the S. R. Sentinel Office.

López de Gomara, F. 1554. *Historia de Mexico*. Port Juan Bellero: Al Salmon.

Lopez, L., S. Langini, S. Fleichman, M. Portela, and C. Ortega Soler. 2001. Iron deficiency in pregnant women with pica. *Journal of the American Dietetic Society* 9: A-104.

Lopez, L., S. Langini, M. Pita de Portela. 2007. Maternal iron status and neonatal outcomes in women with pica during pregnancy. *International Journal of Gynaecology and Obstetrics* 98: 151–52.

Lotan, N., S. Siderman, A. Tabak, U. Taitelman, H. Mihich, and S. Lupovich. 1983. In vivo evaluation of a composite sorbent for the treatment of paraquat intoxication by hemoperfusion. *International Journal of Artificial Organs* 6: 207–13.

Lourie, R. S. 1971. Prevention of lead paint—or prevention of pica? *Pediatrics* 48: 490–91.

Loveland, C. J., T. H. Furst, G. C. Lauritzen. 1989. Geophagia in human populations. *Food and Foodways* 3: 333–56.

Lowry, L. K., D. C. Cherry, C. F. Brady, B. Huggins, A. M. D'Sa, and J. L. Levin. 2004. An unexplained case of elevated blood lead in a Hispanic child. *Environmental Health Perspectives* 112: 222–25.

Lundberg, J., D. A. McFarlane, R. S. Harmon, C. M. Wicks, D. Ford, W. B. White. 2006. Speleogenesis of the Mount Elgon elephant caves, Kenya. In *Perspectives on Karst geomorphology, hydrology, and geochemistry: A tribute volume to Derek C. Ford and William B. White*, 51–63.

Luoba, A., P. Geissler, B. Estambale, J. Ouma, D. Alusala, R. Ayah et al. 2005. Earth-eating and reinfection with intestinal helminths among pregnant and lactating women in western Kenya. *Tropical Medicine and International Health* 10: 220–27.

MacClancy, J. 2007. Earthy realism: Geophagy in literature and art. In J. MacClancy, H. MacBeth, and J. Henry, eds., *Consuming the Inedible: Cross-disciplinary approaches*, 224–33. New York: Berghahn Books.

Madden, L. J. 1998. Pica and eptides: Assessing gastrointestinal malaise. Ph.D. diss., University of Washington.

Mahaney, W. C. 1987. Notes and records: Behavior of the African buffalo on Mount Kenya. *African Journal of Ecology* 25: 199–202.

Mahaney, W., R. Hancock, and M. Inoue. 1993. Geochemistry and clay mineralogy of soils eaten by Japanese macaques. *Primates* 34: 85–91.

Mahaney, W., M. Milner, S. Aufreiter, R. Hancock, R. Wrangham, and S. Campbell S. 2005. Soils consumed by chimpanzees of the Kanyawara community in the Kibale Forest, Uganda. *International Journal of Primatology* 26: 1375–98.

Mahaney, W. C., M. W. Milner, M. Hs, R. Hancock, S. Aufreiter, M. Reich et al. 2000. Mineral and chemical analyses of soils eaten by humans in Indonesia. *International Journal of Environmental Health Research* 10: 93–109.

Malenganisho, W., P. Magnussen, B. J. Vennervald, H. Krarup, P. Kaestel, J. Siza et al. 2007. Intake of alcoholic beverages is a predictor of iron status and hemoglobin in adult Tanzanians. *Journal of Nutrition* 137: 2140–46.

Maler, E. C. F. 1692. *Disputatio medica inauguralis de pica.* Basileae: Typis Joh. Rudolphi Genathii.

Mallory, W. H. 1926. *China: Land of famine.* New York: American Geographical Society.

Mansfield, F. 1977. Investigation of pica in Pitt County, North Carolina. MS thesis, East Carolina University, Greenville.

Marchi, M., and P. Cohen. 1990. Early childhood eating behaviors and adolescent eating disorders. *Journal of the American Academy of Child and Adolescent Psychiatry* 29: 112–17.

Marco Polo/Bartoli, A., and A. D. White. 1863. *I viaggi di Marco Polo.* Firenze: F. Le Monnier.

Marriott, A. 1948. *María, the potter of San Ildefonso.* Norman: U of Oklahoma P.

Martel, Y. 2001. *Life of Pi.* New York: Harcourt.

Martini, and Grothe. 1910. Ueber essbare Erden und ihre Verwendung als Heilmittel. *Deutsche Medizinische Wochenschrift* 36: 900.

Mascolo, N., V. Summa, and F. Tateo. 2004. In vivo experimental data on the mobility of hazardous chemical elements from clays. *Applied Clay Science* 25: 23–28.

Mason, D. 1833. On Atrophia a Ventriculo (mal d'Estomac), or dirt-eating. *Edinburgh Medical and Surgical Journal* 39: 289–96.

Mattson, D. J., G. I. Green, and R. Swalley. 1999. Geophagy by Yellowstone grizzly bears. *Ursus* 11: 109–16.

Maupetit. 1911 (Apr.). Le géophagisme au Laos Siamois. *Bulletin de la Société médico-chirurgicale de l'Indochine*: 176–81.

Maxwell, J. 1835. Pathological inquiry into the nature of cachexia Africana. *Jamaica Physical Journal* 2: 409–35.

Mbati-Mwaka, M. 1993. Prevalence of pica consumption among pregnant women from lower and higher economic groups. MS thesis, University of Nairobi (Kenya).

McAlpine, C., and N. N. Singh. 1986. Pica in institutionalized mentally retarded persons. *Journal of Mental Deficiency Research* 30: 171–78.

Mccaffrey, R. J. 1985. Appropriateness of kaolin consumption as an index of motion sickness in the rat. *Physiology and Behavior* 35: 151–56.

McDonald, R., and S. R. Marshall. 1964. The value of iron therapy in pica. *Pediatrics* 34: 558–62.

McElnay, J., H. Mukhtar, P. D'Arcy, D. Temple, and P. Collier. 1982. The effect of magnesium trisilicate and kaolin on the in vivo absorption of chloroquine. *Journal of Tropical Medicine and Hygiene* 85: 159–63.

McIlwaine, S. 1939. *The southern poor-white from Lubberland to Tobacco Road.* Norman: U of Oklahoma P.

McIntyre, P. 2000. "That Dirt Was Good!": Memories of geophagy among Alabama Black Belt tenant farmers. *Tributaries* 3: 59–74.

McLoughlin, I. 1988. Pica as a cause of death in three mentally handicapped men. *British Journal of Psychiatry* 152: 842–45.

Mérat, F. V., and A. J. de Lens. 1834. *Dictionnaire universel de matière médicale et de thérapeutique générale; contenant l'indication, la description et l'emploi de tous les médicamens connus dans les diverses parties du globe.* Paris: J.-B. Baillière, Méquignon-Marvis.

Merkatz, I. R. 1961. Parotid enlargement resulting from excessive ingestion of starch. *New England Journal of Medicine* 265: 1304–1306.

Meyer, P., T. Pivetz, T. Dignam, D. Homa, J. Schoonover, D. Brody. 2003. Surveillance for elevated blood lead levels among children—United States, 1997–2001. *MMWR Surveillance summaries: Morbidity and mortality weekly report* 52: 1–21.

Michaelis, J., and H. Boezo. 1638. *Disputatio medica inauguralis de pica.* Lipsiae/Leipzig: Typis haered. Frid. Lanckisch.

Mikkelsen, T. B., A. M. Andersen, and S. F. Olsen. 2006. Pica in pregnancy in a privileged population: Myth or reality. *Acta Obstetricia et Gynecologica Scandinavica* 85: 1265–66.

Millican, F. K., E. M. Layman, R. S. Lourie, L. Y. Takahashi, and C. C. Dublin. 1962. The prevalence of ingestion and mouthing of nonedible substances by children. *Clinical Proceedings of the Children's Hospital of District of Columbia* 18: 207–14.

Millot, G. 1979. Clay. *Scientific American* 240: 109–18.

Minnich, V., A. Okcuoglu, Y. Tarcon, A. Arcasoy, S. Cin, O. Yorukoglu et al. 1968. Pica in Turkey. II. Effect of clay upon iron absorption. *American Journal of Clinical Nutrition* 21: 78–86.

Mitchell, D., C. Wells, N. Hoch, K. Lind, S. Woods, and L. Mitchell. 1976. Poison induced pica in rats. *Physiology and Behavior* 17: 691–97.

Mitra, S. C. 1904. Note on clay eating as a racial characteristic. *Anthropological Society of Bombay* 7: 284–91.

Mohaghegh, M. 1976. The title of a work of Razi with reference to al-Tin al-Nishaburi. In *The First International Symposium for the History of Arabic Science,* 338–40. Aleppo, Syria: Institute for the History of Arabic Science.

Mohan, M., K. Agarwal, I. Bhutt, and P. Khanduja. 1968. Iron therapy in pica. *Journal of the Indian Medical Association* 51: 16–18.

Moore, K. L., and T. V. N. Persaud. 1998. *The developing human: Clinically oriented embryology.* Philadelphia: Saunders.

More, J., F. Benazet, J. Fioramonti, and M. T. Droy-Lefaix. 1987. Effects of treatment with smectite on gastric and intestinal glycoproteins in the rat: A histochemical study. *Histochemical Journal* 19: 665–70.

Morel-Fatio, A., and A. Tobler. 1896. Comer Barro. In *Mélanges de philologie romane dédiés à Carl Wahlund à l'occasion du cinquantième anniversaire de sa naissance (7 janvier 1896),* 41–49. Macon: Protat Frères, Imprimeurs.

Morrison, T. 1987. *Song of Solomon.* New York: Plume.

Morrison, T. 1998. *Paradise.* New York: Knopf.

Moss, J, M. Nissenblatt, and T. Inul. 1974. Letter: Successive picas. *Annals of Internal Medicine* 80: 425.

Motherby, G. 1785. *A new medical dictionary, or, General repository of physic: Containing an explanation of the terms and a description of the various particulars relating to anatomy, physiology, physic, surgery, materia medica, chemistry, &c.* London: J. Johnson.

Muccius, J., and N. Hartmannus. 1606. *Disputatio physica De pica seu malacia.* Lipsiae: Abrahamus Lamberg imprimebat.

Muller, J. B. 1722. Description of the Ostiacks, a Nation in Siberia. In F. C. Weber, ed., The present state of Russia In two volumes Being an account of the government of that country, both civil and ecclesiastical; of the Czar's forces by sea and land The whole being the journal of a foreign minister who resided in Russia at that time, 42–60. London: Printed for W. Taylor. W. and J. Innys, and J. Osborn.

Murdock, G. P., and D. R. White. 1969. Standard Cross-Cultural Sample. *Ethnology* 9: 329–69.

Mycyk, M.B., and J. B. Leikin. 2004. Combined exchange transfusion and chelation therapy for neonatal lead poisoning. *Annals of Pharmacotherapy* 38: 821–24.

National Research Council and the Institute of Medicine. 2007. *Earth materials and health: Research priorities for earth science and public health.* Washington, D.C.: National Academies Press.

Nchito, M., P. W. Geissler, L. Mubila, H. Friis, A. Olsen. 2004. Effects of iron and multimicronutrient supplementation on geophagy: A two-by-two factorial study among Zambian schoolchildren in Lusaka. *Transactions of the Royal Society of Tropical Medicine and Hygiene* 98: 218–27.

Nyaruhucha, C. N. 2009. Food cravings, aversions and pica among pregnant women in Dar es Salaam, Tanzania. *Tanzanian Journal of Health Research* 11: 29–34.

Ofoefule, S. I., and M. Okonta. 1999. Adsorption studies of ciprofloxacin: Evaluation of magnesium trisilicate, kaolin and starch as alternatives for the management of ciprofloxacin poisoning. *Bollettino Chimico Farmaceutica* 138: 239–42.

Oke, O. L. 1972. Rickets in developing countries. *World Review of Nutrition and Dietetics* 15: 86–103.

Okonek, S., H. Setyadharma, A. Borchert, and E. G. Krienke. 1982. Activated charcoal is as effective as fuller's earth or bentonite in paraquat poisoning. *Klinische Wochenschrift* 60: 207–10.

Olynyk, F., and D. Sharpe. 1982. Mercury poisoning in paper pica. *New England Journal of Medicine* 306: 1056–57.

Oribasius, U. C. Bussemaker, C. V. Daremberg, and A. Molinier. 1851. *Oeuvres d'Oribase, texte Grec, en grande partie inédit, collationnée sur les manuscrits.* Paris: Impr. nationale.

O'Rourke, D. E., J. G. Quinn, J. O. Nicholson, and H. H. Gibson. 1967. Geophagia during pregnancy. *Obstetrics and Gynecology* 29: 581–84.

Osman, A. K. 1985. Dietary practices and aversions during pregnancy and lactation among Sudanese women. *Journal of Tropical Pediatrics* 31: 16–20.

Osman, Y., Y. Wali, and O. Osman. 2005. Craving for ice and iron-deficiency anemia: A case series from Oman. *Pediatric Hematology and Oncology* 22: 127–31.

Oyeyemi, H. 2009. *White is for witching.* New York: Nan A. Talese/Doubleday.

Palahniuk, C. 1999. *Survivor: A novel.* New York: Anchor Books.

Pallas, P. S. 1776. *Samlungen historischer nachrichten über die mongolischen völkerschaften.* St. Petersburg: Kanserlichen Akademie der Wissenschaften.

Paulus Aegineta/F. Adams. 1844. *The seven books of Paulus Aegineta, tr. from the Greek, with a commentary embracing a complete view of the knowledge possessed by the Greeks, Romans, and Arabians on all subjects connected with medicine and surgery.* London: Sydenham Society.

Payton, E., E. P. Crump, and C. P. Horton. 1960. Growth and development VII: Dietary habits of 571 pregnant southern Negro women. *Journal of the American Dietetic Society* 37: 129–36.

Peirce, R. 1697. *Bath memoirs: or, observations in three and forty years practice, at the Bath what cures have been there wrought.* Bristol: H. Hammond.

Pelto, G. H., A. H. Goodman, and D. L. Dufour. 2000. The biocultural perspective in nutritional anthropology. In A. H. Goodman, D. L. Dufour, and G. H. Pelto, eds., *Nutritional Anthropology,* 1–9. Mountain View, Calif.: Mayfield.

Perry, M. C. 1977. Cautopyreiophagia. *New England Journal of Medicine* 296: 824.

Phillips, U. B. 1929. *Life and Labor in the Old South.* Boston: Little, Brown.

Pliny/Rackham, H. T. 1952. *Natural history.* Cambridge: Harvard UP.

Ploss, H. H., M. Bartels, P. R. A. Bartels, and E. J. Dingwall. 1938. *Woman: An historical gynæcological and anthropological compendium.* St. Louis: C.V. Mosby.

Posner, L. B., C. M. Mccottry, A. C. Posner. 1957. Pregnancy craving and pica. *Obstetrics and Gynecology* 9: 270–72.

Post-Dispatch (St. Louis). 1902. Seventy-five St. Louisans Eat Dirt. *Current Literature* 32: 568–70.

Prasad, A. S. 1996. Zinc deficiency in women, infants, and children. *Journal of the American College of Nutrition* 15: 113–20.

Prasad, A., J. A. Halsted, and M. Nadimi. 1961. Syndrome of iron deficiency anemia, hepatosplenomegaly, hypogonadism, dwarfism and geophagia. *American Journal of Medicine* 31: 532–46.

Prasad, A., A. Miale, Z. Farid, H. H. Sandstead, and A. R. Schulbert. 1963. Zinc metabolism in patients with the syndrome of iron deficiency anemia, hepatosplenomegaly, dwarfism, and hypognadism. *Journal of Laboratory and Clinical Medicine* 61: 537–49.

Prince, L. B. 1915. *Spanish mission churches of New Mexico.* Cedar Rapids, Iowa: Torch Press.

Profet, M. 1992. Pregnancy sickness as adaptation: A deterrent to maternal ingestion of teratogens. In J. H. Barkow, L. Cosmides, and J. Tooby, eds., *The adapted mind: Evolutionary psychology and the generation of culture,* 327–66. New York: Oxford UP.

Puckett, N. N. 1926. *Folk beliefs of the southern Negro.* Chapel Hill: U of North Carolina P; London: Milford.

Rainville, A. J. 1998. Pica practices of pregnant women are associated with lower maternal hemoglobin level at delivery. *Journal of the American Dietetic Society* 98: 293–96.

Reading, S. M. 1982. An ethnography: The health beliefs of Sioux Native Americans living in the Denver urban area. Master's thesis, University of Colorado, Boulder.

Reid, R. M. 1992. Cultural and medical perspectives on geophagia. *Medical Anthropology* 13: 337–51.

Reinbacher, W. R. 2002. *Healing Earths the Third Leg of Medicine: A History of Minerals in Medicine.* 1st Books Library.

Reynolds, R., H. Binder, M. Miller, W. Chang, S. Horan. 1968. Pagophagia and iron deficiency anemia. *Annals of Internal Medicine* 69: 435–40.

Richardson, C. 2002 (Feb. 11). Doc's RX: Ounce of prevention 50-year crusade for healthy living targeted starch, dye and sugar. *New York Daily News,* NY Local.

Richardson, J. 1851. *Arctic searching expedition: a journal of a boat voyage through Rupert's Land and the Arctic Sea, in search of the discovery ships under command of Sir John Franklin. With an appendix on the physical geography of North America.* London: Longman, Brown, Green, and Longmans.

Riverius, L., N. Culpeper, and A. Cole. 1663. *The practice of physick wherein is plainly set forth the nature, cause, differences, and several sorts of signs: Together with the cure of all diseases in the body of man. With many additions in several places never printed before. In twenty-four books.* London: Printed by Peter Cole, printer and bookseller, at the sign of the Printing-press in Cornhil near the Royal Exchange.

Robbins, T. 1984. *Jitterbug perfume.* Toronto and New York: Bantam.

Robertson, R. H. S. 1986. *Fuller's earth: A history of calcium montmorillonite.* Hythe, Kent, UK: Volturna Press.

Robinson, B. A, W. Tolan, and O. Golding-Beecher. 1990. Childhood pica: Some aspects of the clinical profile in Manchester, Jamaica. *West Indian Medical Journal* 39: 20–26.

Rogers, M. E. 1972. Practice of pica among iron deficient pregnant women. MS thesis, Auburn University, Auburn, Alabama.

Rokni, S. 1990. Assessment of the nutritional status of children 13–60 months living in rural areas of Sirjon County, Iran. MS thesis, California State University, Long Beach.

Romer, B., F. X. Grollig, and H. B. Haley. 1976. The use of argillaceous earth as medicament. In *Medical Anthropology,* 269–77. The Hague: Mouton.

Roosendaal, J. J., and J. J. Weits-Binnerts. 1997. [Aspects of pica in adult psychiatric patients]. *Nederlands Tijdschrift voor Geneeskunde* 141: 306–307.

Root-Bernstein, R. S., and M. Root-Bernstein. 1997. *Honey, mud, maggots, and other medical marvels: The science behind folk remedies and old wives' tales.* Boston: Houghton Mifflin.

Roselle, H. 1970. Association of laundry starch and clay ingestion with anemia in New York City. *Archives of Internal Medicine* 125: 57–61.

Rosner, D., and G. Markowitz. 1985. A "gift of God"?: The public health controversy over leaded gasoline during the 1920s. *American Journal of Public Health* 75: 344–52.

Roth, E. A. 2004. *Culture, biology, and anthropological demography.* Cambridge: Cambridge UP.

Roth, W. E., and R. Etheridge. 1897. *Ethnological studies among the north-west-central Queensland aborigines.* Brisbane: E. Gregory, Government Printer.

Roughley, T. 1823. *The Jamaica planter's guide, or, A system for planting and managing a sugar estate, or other plantations in that island and throughout the British West Indies in general.* London: Printed for Longman, Hurst, Rees, Orme, and Brown.

Rowles-Sewing, S. 1981. "We're made from clay, it won't hurt nobody": A cross-cultural study of geophagia in Houston. MA thesis, University of Houston, Houston.

Ruby, M. V., A. Davis, R. Schoof, and S. Eberle. 1996. Estimation of lead and arsenic bioavailability using a physiologically based extraction test. *Environmental Science & Technology* 30: 422–30.

Ruddock, J. C. 1924. Lead poisoning in children: With special reference to pica. *Journal of the American Medical Association* 82: 1682–84.

Rutherford, D.G., and W. L. Distant. 1881. Notes on the people of Batanga. *Journal of the Anthropological Institute of Great Britain and Ireland* 10: 463–70.

Saathoff, E., A. Olsen, J. D. Kvalsvig, and P. W. Geissler. 2002. Geophagy and its association with geohelminth infection in rural schoolchildren from northern KwaZulu-Natal, South Africa. *Transactions of the Royal Society of Tropical Medicine and Hygiene* 96: 485–90.

Sage, J. C. 1962. The practice, incidence and effect of starch eating on Negro women at Temple University Medical Center. MS thesis, Temple University, Philadelphia.

Salmon, W. 1691. *Pharmacopoeia Londinensis, or, The new London dispensatory in VI books, translated into English for the publick good, and fitted to the whole art of healing.* London: Printed for T. Bassett, R. Chiswell, M. Wotton, G. Conyers, A. and I. Dawks, and are to be sold by Awnsham and John Churchill.

Say, B., S. Ozsoylu, and I. Berkel. 1969. Geophagia associated with iron-deficiency anemia, hepatosplenomegaly, hypogonadism and dwarfism: A syndrome probably associated with zinc deficiency. *Clinical Pediatrics* 8: 661–68.

Sayers, G., D. Lipschitz, M. Sayers, H. Sefterl, T. Bothwell, and R. Charlton. 1974. Relationship between pica and iron nutrition in Johannesburg Black adults. *South African Medical Journal* 48: 1655–60.

Schmidt, C. 1871. Essbare erden aus Lappland und Sud-Persien. *Bulletin de l'Académie impérial des sciences de St Pétersbourg* 14: 203–207.

Schwab, E. B., and M. L. Axelson. 1984. Dietary changes of pregnant women: Compulsions and modifications. *Ecology of Food and Nutrition* 14: 143–52.

Severance, H. W., T. Holt, N. Patrone, and L. Chapman. 1988. Profound muscle weakness and hypokalemia due to clay ingestion. *Southern Medical Journal* 81: 272–74.

Shadwell, T. 1691. *The scourers, a comedy: Acted by Their Majesties servants.* London: Printed for James Knapton.

Shannon, R. 1794. *Practical observations on the operation and effects of certain medicines in the prevention and cure of diseases to which Europeans are subject in hot climates, . . . applicable also to the prevention and cure of the scurvy . . . and Observations on the Diseases and Diet of Negroes . . . With a copious explanatory index.* London: Printed for the author and sold by Vernor and Hood.

Sharlet, J. 2002. *I Ate Dirt* (*see* http://killingthebuddha.com/mag/dispatch/i-ate-dirt/). Accessed July 21, 2009.

Sharp-Ross, M. L. 1987. Geophagy and amylophagy in pregnancy in Mobile, Alabama. MA thesis, Louisiana State University.

Sherman, P. 1988. The levels of analysis. *Animal Behavior* 36: 616–19.

Sherman, P. 1989. The clitoris debate and the levels of analysis. *Animal Behavior* 37: 697–98.

Silverman, M., and R. Perkins. 1966. Bilateral parotid enlargement and starch ingestion. *Annals of Internal Medicine* 75: 842–46.

Simon, S. L. 1998. Soil ingestion by humans: A review of history, data, and etiology with application to risk assessment of radioactively contaminated soil. *Health Physics* 74: 647–72.

Simpson, E., J. Mull, E. Longley, and J. East. 2000. Pica during pregnancy in low-income women born in Mexico. *Western Journal of Medicine* 173: 20–24.

Sinclair, M. C. 1957. *Southern belle.* New York: Crown.

Singhi, S., R. Ravishanker, P. Singhi, and R. Nath. 2003. Low plasma zinc and iron in pica. *Indian Journal of Pediatrics* 70: 139–43.

Skog, K. 1993. Cooking procedures and food mutagens: A literature review. *Food and Chemical Toxicology* 31: 655–75.

Smith, B., B. Rawlins, M. Cordeiro, M. Hutchins, J. Tiberindwa, I. L. Sserunjog et al. 2000. The bioaccessibility of essential and potentially toxic trace elements in tropical soils from Mukono District, Uganda. *Journal of the Geological Society* 157: 885–91.

Smith, J. C., and J. A. Halsted. 1970. Clay ingestion (geophagia) as a source of zinc for rats. *Journal of Nutrition* 100: 973–80.

Smulian, J., S. Motiwala, and R. Sigman. 1995. Pica in a rural obstetric population. *Southern Medical Journal* 88: 1236–40.

Snowdon, C. 1977. A nutritional basis for lead pica. *Physiology and Behavior* 18: 885–93.

Solyom, C., L. Solyom, and R. Freeman. 1991. An unusual case of pica. *Canadian Journal of Psychiatry* 36: 50–53.

Sontag, C., A. Kettaneh, O. Fain, V. Eclache, M. Thomas. 2001. [Rapid regression of prolonged pagophagia after treatment of iron deficiency]. *La Presse Médicale* 30: 321–23.

Soranus. 1956. *Gynecology*. Baltimore: Johns Hopkins UP.

Speer, S. J. 1980. The relationship of pagophagia and iron deficiency anemia in pregnant women. MS thesis, Texas Woman's University, Denton.

Speirs, J., and R. Jacobson. 1976. [The consumption of ice as a symptom of iron deficiency]. *South African Medical Journal* 50: 1742.

Spence, K. 1993 (Apr. 10). In search of the good earth. *Financial Times*. Travel sec., 17.

Spencer, T. 2002 (Jan. 25). *Dirt-eating persists in rural south*. Newhouse News Service (*see* www.newhouse.com/archive/story1c012502.html). Accessed Dec. 19, 2006.

Staszewski, J. 1963. Population distribution according to the climate areas of W. Koppen. *Professional Geographer* 15: 12–15.

Steinbeck, J. 1967 [1939]. *The grapes of wrath*. Garden City, N.Y: International Collectors Library.

Steinbeck, J. 2002 [1952]. *East of Eden*. New York: Penguin Books.

Stevens, P. 1993. "Pica." Nursing RSA 8: 40.

Stevenson, M. C. 1908. *Thirtieth annual report of the Bureau of American Ethnology: Ethnobotany of the Zuni Indians*. Washington, D.C.: GPO.

Stoltzfus, R. 2001. Defining iron-deficiency anemia in public health terms: A time for reflection. *Journal of Nutrition* 131: 565S–567S.

Stoltzfus, R. J., and M. L. Dreyfuss. 1998. *Guidelines for the use of iron supplements to prevent and treat iron deficiency anemia*. Washington, D.C.: ILSI Press.

Stoltzfus, R., M. Dreyfuss, H. Chwaya, and M. Albonico. 1997. Hookworm control as a strategy to prevent iron deficiency. *Nutrition Reviews* 55: 223–32.

Strose, K., and H. Suhle. 1891. Mitteilung uber das Diatomeenlager bei Klieken in Anhalt. In *IX Jahresbericht des Friedrichs-Realgymnasiums und der Vorschule des Fridericianum fur das Schuljahr 1890–1891*, 1–7.

Struhsaker, T. T., D. O. Cooney, and K. S. Siex. 1997. Charcoal consumption by Zanzibar Red Colobus monkeys: Its function and its ecological and demographic consequences. *International Journal of Primatology* 18: 61–72.

Sudilovsky, J. 2007. *Catholic News Service*: Bethlehem's Milk Grotto brings faith, hope and sometimes babies (*see* www.catholicnews.com/data/stories/cns/0707062.htm). Accessed July 20, 2009.

Sule, S., and H. N. Madugu. 2001. Pica in pregnant women in Zaria, Nigeria. *Nigerian Journal of Medicine* 10: 25–27.

Suttles G. 1968. *The social order of the slum: Ethnicity and territory in the inner city*. Chicago and London: U of Chicago P.

Swerdlow, J. 2000 (Apr.). Nature's RX. *National Geographic*: 98–100.

Szajewska, H., P. Dziechciarz, and J. Mrukowicz. 2006. Meta-analysis: Smectite in the treatment of acute infectious diarrhoea in children. *Alimentary Pharmacology & Therapeutics* 23: 217–27.

Takeda, N., S. Hasegawa, M. Morita, and T. Matsunaga. 1993. Pica in rats is analogous to emesis: An animal model in emesis research. *Phamacology, Biochemistry, and Behavior* 45: 817–21.

Talkington, K. M., N. F. Gant, D. E. Scott, and J. A. Pritchard. 1970. Effect of ingestion of starch and some clays on iron absorption. *American Journal of Obstetrics and Gynecology* 108: 262–67.

Tandu-Umba, N., and M. Paluku. 1988. Risque nutrionnel de la population obstetricale aux cliniques universitaires de Kinshasa. *Médicine et nutrition* 24: 178–80.

Tanis, A. L. 1955. Lead poisoning in children; including nine cases treated with edathamil calcium-disodium. *American Journal of Diseases of Children* 89: 325–31.

Tayie, F. A. K, and A. Lartey. 1999. Pica practice among pregnant Ghanaians: Relationship with infant birth weight and maternal haemoglobin level. *Ghana Medical Journal* 33: 67–76.

Taylor, S. H. 1979. Prevalence of earth and laundry starch consumption during pregnancy. MA thesis, University of Texas, Houston.

Telford, W. 1822. On the Mal d'Estomac. *Medical and Physical Journal* (London) 47: 450–58.

Thibault de Chanvalon, J. 1761. *Voyage à la Martinique: Contenant diverses observations sur la physique l'histoire naturelle, l'agriculture, les moeœurs, & les usages de cette isle, faites en 1751 & dans les années suivantes.* Paris: J. B. Bauche.

Thomas, F. B., J. M. Falko, and K. Zuckerman. 1976. Inhibition of intestinal iron absorption by laundry starch. *Gastroenterology* 71: 1028–32.

Thomas, R. W. B. 1978. Pica and folkdrug use in pregnancy. MS thesis, University of Virginia, Charlottesville.

Thompson, C. J. S. 1914. Terra Sigillata, a famous medicament of ancient times. *Transactions of the 17th International Medical Conference*, Sec. 23: 433–44.

Thompson, W. T. 1852. *Chronicles of Pineville*. Philadelphia: Getz and Buck.

Thomson, J. 1997. Anaemia in pregnant women in eastern Caprivi, Namibia. *South African Medical Journal* 87: 1544–47.

Thorndike, L. 1923. *A history of magic and experimental science*. London: Macmillan.

Torrette, M. 1836. Missions des Lazaristes en Chine. *Annales de la Propagation de la Foi* 48: 57–87.

Tozer, H. F. 1890. *The islands of the Aegean*. Oxford: Clarendon Press.

Urban Dictionary. 2009. Dirt (*see* www.urbandictionary.com/define.php?term=dirt). Accessed July 8, 2009.

Vermeer, D. E. 1966. Geophagy among the Tiv of Nigeria. *Annals of the Association of American Geographers* 56: 197–204.

Vermeer, D. E. 1971. Geophagy among the Ewe of Ghana. *Ethnology* 10: 56–72.

Vermeer, D. E., and D. A. Frate. 1975. Geophagy in a Mississippi County. *Annals of the Association of American Geographers* 65: 414–25.

Vermeer, D., and D. Frate. 1979. Geophagia in rural Mississippi: Environmental and cultural contexts and nutritional implications. *American Journal of Clinical Nutrition* 32: 2129–35.

Vernon, O. 2003. *Eden.* New York: Grove Press.

Von Bonsdorff, B. 1977. Pica: A hypothesis. *British Journal of Haematology* 35.3: 476–77.

Von Humboldt, A., A. Bonpland, H. M. Williams. 1821. *Personal narrative of travels to the equinoctial regions of the new continent during the years 1799–1804.* Vol. 5. Paris: Longman, Hurst, Rees, Orme, and Brown [etc.].

Wakou, B. A. N. 2003. *Consumption of clay, herbs and alcohol by women of childbearing age in Kampala, Uganda.* Ph.D. diss., Oklahoma State University, Stillwater.

Walker, A., B. Walker, J. Jones, M. Verardi, and C. Walker. 1985. Nausea and vomiting and dietary cravings and aversions during pregnancy in South African women. *British Journal of Obstetrics and Gynaecology* 92: 484–89.

Ward, P., and N. G. Kutner. 1999. Reported pica behavior in a sample of incident dialysis patients. *Journal of Renal Nutrition* 9: 14–20.

Warshauer, S. 1966. Starch-eater's anemia. *Southern Medical Journal* 59: 538–40.

Weiss-Amer, M. 1993. Medieval women's guides to food during pregnancy: Origins, texts, and traditions. *Canadian Bulletin of Medical History* 10: 5–23.

Welch, R. 2008. *South Carolina—Origin of the term sandlapper* (*see* www.sciway. net/hist/sandlapper.html). Accessed June 25, 2009.

Whiting, A. F. 1939. *Ethnobotany of the Hopi.* Flagstaff: Museum of Northern Arizona.

Whiting, A. N. 1947. Clay, starch, and soot eating among southern rural Negroes in North Carolina. *Journal of Negro Education* 16: 610–12.

Wikipedia. 2009. *Salad Fingers.* (*see* http://en.wikipedia.org/wiki/Salad_fingers). Accessed Jan. 2010.

Wilensky-Lanford, E. 2005 (Sept. 5). A corner of Kyrgyzstan has a cure-all: Let them eat clay. *New York Times,* A5.

Wiley, A. S. 1992. Adaptation and the biocultural paradigm in medical anthropology: A critical review. *Medical Anthropology Quarterly* 6: 216–36.

Wiley, A. S., and S. H. Katz. 1998. Geophagy in pregnancy: A test of a hypothesis. *Current Anthropology* 39: 532–45.

Wilks, C. S. 1974. Cultural transmission of exotic health practices. Ph.D. diss., St. Louis University.

Williamson, J. 1817. *Medical and miscellaneous observations, relative to the West India Islands.* Edinburgh: Smellie.

Wilson, M. 2003. Clay mineralogical and related characteristics of geophagic materials. *Journal of Chemical Ecology* 29: 1525–47.

Wong, M. S., D. A. Bundy, and M. H. Golden. 1991. The rate of ingestion of *Ascaris lumbricoides* and *Trichuris trichiura* eggs in soil and its relationship to infection in two children's homes in Jamaica. *Transactions of the Royal Society of Tropical Medicine and Hygiene* 85: 89–91.

Woods, S. C., and R. S. Weisinger. 1970. Pagophagia in the albino rat. *Science* 169: 1334–36.

World Health Organization. 1993. *The ICD-10 classification of mental and behavioural disorders: Diagnostic criteria for research.* Geneva: World Health Organization.

Wrenn, K. 1989. Fecal impaction due to geophagia. *Southern Medical Journal* 82: 932.

Wyllie, J.A. Oct. 1, 1909. Alleged slavery in St. Thomé. *London Times (Weekly Edition)*: 629.

Yang, S., W. Hoo, and C. A. J. Sainson. 1904. *Nan-tchao ye-che . . . Histoire particulière du Nantchao.* Paris: Imprimerie nationale, E. Leroux.

Yetts, W. P. 1919. Taoist Tales. *New China Review* 1: 11–18.

Youdim, M. B., and T. C. Iancu. 1977. Pica hypothesis. *British Journal of Haematology* 36: 298.

Young, S. L. 2002. Critically ecological medical anthropology: Selecting and applying theory to anemia during pregnancy on Pemba, Zanzibar. *Medische Anthropologie* 14: 321–52.

Young, S. L. 2010. Pica in pregnancy: New ideas about an old condition. *Annual Review of Nutrition* 30: 403–422.

Young, S. L., D. Goodman, T. Farag, S. Ali, M. Khatib, S. Khalfan et al. 2007. Geophagia is not associated with Trichuris or hookworm transmission in Zanzibar, Tanzania. *Transactions of the Royal Society of Tropical Medicine and Hygiene* 101: 766–72.

Young, S. L., S. Khalfan, T. Farag, T. Kavle, S. Ali, H. Hamad et al. 2010a. Pica is associated with anemia and gastrointestinal distress among pregnant Zanzibari women. *American Journal of Tropical Medicine & Hygiene* 83: 144–51.

Young, S. L., and G. H. Pelto. 2006. Core concepts in nutritional anthropology. In N. J. Temple, T. Wilson, and D. R. Jacobs, eds., *Nutritional Health: Strategies for Disease Prevention*, 425–37. Totowa, N.J.: Humana Press.

Young, S. L., M. J. Wilson, S. Hillier, E. Delbos, S. M. Ali, and R. Stoltzfus. 2010b. Differences and commonalities in physical, chemical, and mineralogical properties of Zanzibari geophagic soils. *Journal of Chemical Ecology* 36: 129–40.

Young, S. L., M. Wilson, D. Miller, S. Hillier. 2008. Toward a comprehensive approach to the collection and analysis of pica substances, with emphasis on geophagic materials. *PLoS ONE* 3: e3147.

Acknowledgments

This book is the product of many minds, and it is a great pleasure to thank each and every one of them. First and foremost, I would like to extend my deep gratitude to the many scholars on whose shoulders I have stood for a better vantage point of pica. This book would not be possible without their laborious research efforts, from antiquity to the present, to identify, describe, and measure both pica behavior and pica substances.

I have been blessed with kind and wise academic mentors who have guided me well as I traversed the sometimes treacherous biocultural terrain: Gretel Pelto, Kathleen Rasmussen, Rebecca Stoltzfus, Paul Sherman, Caroline Chantry, and Sjaak van der Geest. Their suggestions and advice have prepared me for a wide range of endeavors, both scientific and personal.

A number of scientists and collaborators in different fields have my unending gratitude for their hard work and patience as I learned to communicate with them about "their" disciplines. In *soil science*: Evelyne Delbos, Stephen Hillier, M. Jeffrey Wilson. *Food science*: Ray Glahn and Dennis Miller. *Parasitology*: Dave Goodman. *Statistics*: Françoise Vermeylen. *Hoodoo*: Catherine Yronwode (luckymojo.com). *Waste management*: Jim McNaughton. *Bayou fishing*: Ripp Blank.

The diligence and attention to detail with which librarians around the world have pursued my requests is deeply appreciated. In particular, Cornell University has a wonderful team of library scientists and staff at the Division of Rare and Manuscript Collections at Kroch Library, Mann Library, the Veterinary Library, Interlibrary Loan Office, Library Annex, and Photocopy Services at Olin Library. I gratefully acknowledge all of them.

I have also been helped by many polyglot friends and colleagues for translations of passages on pica: Jen Baker, Maurits Barendrecht, Benedetta Bartali, Urvashi

Batra, David Caroline, Brian English, Tamer Farag, Tim Haupt, Damarys Hernandez, Jacqueline Kung'u, Helena Pachon, Rinat Ran-Ressler, Angelos Sidakalis, Owen Strijland, Vincenzo Vitelli, and Winthrop "Skip" Wetherbee. I also appreciate the many people who have sent me pica clippings, samples, and references over the years: Laura Anderson, Avril Armstrong, Brian Chabot, Gerald Deas, John Dominy, Lia Fernald, Chris Golden, Vivian Hoffman, Lou Grivetti, Rebecca Heidkamp, Ruth Kutalek, Jef Leroy, Nkosi Mbuya, Purnima Menon, Monique Borgerhoff Mulder, Christina Nyhus, Eline Rupert, Trevor Stokes, Lucy Thairu, Roy Thomas, Andrea Wiley, Robin Young, and Stacey Young.

The scientific prowess, kindness, patience, and good humor of many Pembans and expats working in Pemba during the Mama na Afya study helped to make that research as informative as it was: Tamer Farag, Hajji Mohammed Hajji, Justine Kavle, Sabra Said Khalfan, Mzee Khatib, Darrell Mast, Mzee Babu Mlinzi, Shufaa Saleh, Buchi Rashid Salum, the Vileo team, and the entire Pemba Public Health Laboratory–Ivo de Carneri. I am deeply grateful for the openness and patience with which Pembans endured my endless questions about pica.

A girl cannot live on academic curiosity alone, and thanks to financial support for my research on pica from the National Institutes of Health, the Thrasher Research Fund, the Robert Wood Johnson Foundation, Sigma Xi, UCMEXUS, and the University of California, Berkeley, Population Center, I didn't have to. I am particularly grateful to the Wenner-Gren Foundation for salary support while I wrote this book. I'm also indebted to the emotional and domestic support my mom, Robin Young, and sister, Stacey Young, provided from afar and during visits to Oakland as I prepared this book.

I am also touched by the friends, family, and colleagues who have been generous with their time and constructive criticism as they read some truly terrible early chapters: Chaele Arkfeld, Emily Dantzer, Lou Grivetti, Jerome Handler, Janice Lin, Marimar McNaughton, Alexis Steinmetz, Tom Struhsaker, Andrea Wiley, Jeff Wilson, Robin Young, and Stacey Young. I am also very grateful to the anonymous reviewers whose considerable efforts to trudge through earlier drafts of the book greatly improved tone, flow, structure, and conciseness of language. Thank you.

I am indebted to Bruce and Kathy Armbruster for their assurance that I had a book in me, and then ensuring it emerged by introducing me to my editor at Columbia University Press, Patrick Fitzgerald. Through a combination of talent, good sense, and good humor, Patrick, together with Bridget Flannery-McCoy and Roy Thomas, helped me to produce that which you are currently reading.

I'm grateful to Stella Lucks, our first young Lucks, who kept me company as I wrote much of this book. Although her growing presence did not incite pica behavior, it did give me a new appreciation for the unique privileges and challenges that pregnant women face, nutritional and otherwise.

And then there is my greatest debt. And that is to Julius Lucks, who has shared in every part of the research for and writing of this book. I am forever grateful for his constructive criticism, creative vision, scientific accuracy, gentle encouragement, and profound love.

Index

Abeyta, Don Bernardo, 51–52, 142, 177
absorption: by ash, 116; by charcoal, 125–26; by clays, 35, 115, 122–23; definition, 174, 183; of micronutrients, 114–18, 137, 142; by starches, 35, 115, 126–27
acid digests, 110, 111
acorn flour, 128, 129
activated charcoal. *See* charcoal
Adam and Eve, 69
adaptation, 22–23, 113, 128; pica as an, 109, 137
adaptive. *See* adaptation; nonadaptive
addiction: and pica substances generally, 14–15; to starch, 10–12, 84
adsorption, 174, 180, 183
Aetius of Amida, 142, 172
aflatoxins, 120
Alabama, pica in, 95, 145, 146, 179, 180
alimentary canal. *See* digestive tract

alkaloids, 120, 180, 185; in wild potatoes, 128–29
Among the Pines (Gilmore), 153
amount consumed. *See* quantity consumed
amylophagy, 7–12; cessation of, 105–106; in Pemba, 94, 132, 134; prevalence of, 12, 143–46; timing of, 134
anemia: association with pica, 59–60, 100, 141, 161–65; description of, 58–59, 100; hookworms and, 63
animals, geophagy among: diverse, 17, 139, 172; domesticated, 109; as evidence of adaptive benefit, 23, 113; primates, 77, 131
antidiarrheal medicine. *See* diarrhea; Kaopectate; Smecta
Argentina: geophagy among pregnant women in, 143; geophagy and anemia in, 161

detoxification: hypothesis, 119–35,
180; mechanisms of, 120–27, 139,
180; of pathogens, 45,120–22, 137,
139; of toxins, 128–31, 137, 139
diarrhea: charcoal in treatment of, 125;
earth in treatment of, 41, 42, 43,
175; and toxins/pathogens, 120,
121, 131, 132. *See also* gastrointestinal distress
diatomaceous earth, 90–91, 174, 184
dietary supplement. *See* supplementation
difficulties of studying pica, 20–21, 24,
83–85
digestive tract: damage to, 65–66; in
vitro model of, 180; physiology
of, 110, 138, 180; protection of,
121–23
Dioscorides, 36, 141, 174–75
disdain of pica. *See* stigma
disgust for pica. *See* stigma
dismissal of pica. *See* stigma
dissertatios, 77, 78, 142
Dominy, Nathan, 180
Don Quixote (Cervantes), 150–51

earth as food: in the Arctic, 91; in
Europe, 89–90; in Haiti, 91, 93; in
Sierra Leone, 91, 93
earth consumption. *See* geophagic
earth; geophagy
East of Eden (Steinbeck), 158
Eden (Vernon), 159–60
effect modification, 85–86, 184
Ellen Foster (Gibbons), 152–53
embarrassment, about pica, xiv, 84–85
England: geophagy among pregnant
women in, 146; geophagy among
slaves in, 153–54; pica in, 99, 158;
terra sigillata in, 119–20
enterotoxins, 120–21
Esquipulas, Guatemala, 48–50, 176,
177

Europe: geophagy among European settlers, 77; geophagy during famine in,
90–91. *See also* entries for individual
countries
evidence, types of, 27–28

Facebook, 13
famine, 90–91, 129, 142
fatality: with anemia, 59; with diarrhea,
121; with geophagy, 71, 72, 73, 90;
with heavy metal poisoning, 61,
120; with obesity, 66
fecal impaction, 65
fertility, earth used to facilitate, 42,
47, 48
Finland, geophagy in, 91
fitness, 22–23
flour, acorn, 128–29; consumption of,
5, 9; mixed with earth, 90–91
food shortage. *See* hunger
forgetting about pica behavior, 84–85,
181
Fossey, Diane, 131
France: geophagy in, 172; pagophagy
in, 12–13, 142
Fuller's earth, 34, 35
future research, 138–39

Galen: influence on Stumpf, 43; terms
for pica, 4, 141; trip to Lemnos,
36–37, 175
gastrointestinal distress: pica during,
131–32, 135; in Pica Literature Database, 29, 129; and toxins/patho-
gens, 43, 121. *See also* diarrhea
gastroliths, 65
geohelminths, 24, 121, 178, 184; and
anemia, 25, 66, 114, 121; *Ascaris*
(roundworm), 63; geophagy as vector of, 25, 62–64, 66, 114, 149
geophagic earth: binding capacity of,
123–25, 127; in literature, 149–60;
Pemban, 6–7; preparation of, 6, 49,